Pathways to Quality Health Care

REWARDING PROVIDER PERFORMANCE

Aligning Incentives in Medicare

Committee on Redesigning Health Insurance Performance Measures,
Payment, and Performance Improvement Programs

Board on Health Care Services

INSTITUTE OF MEDICINE
OF THE NATIONAL ACADEMIES

THE NATIONAL ACADEMIES PRESS
Washington, D.C.
www.nap.edu

THE NATIONAL ACADEMIES PRESS   500 Fifth Street, N.W.   Washington, DC 20001

This study was supported by Contract No. HHSM-500-2004-00005C between the National Academy of Sciences and U.S. Department of Health and Human Services through the Centers for Medicare and Medicaid Services. Any opinions, findings, conclusions, or recommendations expressed in this publication are those of the author(s) and do not necessarily reflect the view of the organizations or agencies that provided support for this project.

Library of Congress Cataloging-in-Publication Data

Rewarding provider performance : aligning incentives in Medicare /
Committee on Redesigning Health Insurance Performance Measures, Payment, and Performance Improvement Programs, Board on Health Care Services.
    p. ; cm. — (Pathways to quality health care)
  Includes bibliographical references and index.
  ISBN-13: 978-0-309-10216-2 (hardback)
  ISBN-10: 0-309-10216-2 (hardback)
  1. Medicare—Finance. 2. Medicare—Quality control. 3.
Medicare—Administration. 4. Incentive awards—United States. 5.
Performance awards—United States. 6. Medical care—United
States—Quality control. I. Institute of Medicine (U.S.). Committee on
Redesigning Health Insurance Performance Measures, Payment, and
Performance Improvement Programs. II. Series.
  [DNLM: 1. Reimbursement, Incentive—organization &
administration—United States. 2. Medicare—organization &
administration. 3. Quality Assurance, Health Care—economics—United
States. 4. Quality Assurance, Health Care—methods—United States. WT
31 R454 2007]
  RA412.3.R49 2007
  368.4'2600973—dc22
                                    2006033904

Additional copies of this report are available from the National Academies Press, 500 Fifth Street, N.W., Lockbox 285, Washington, DC 20055; (800) 624-6242 or (202) 334-3313 (in the Washington metropolitan area); Internet, http://www. nap.edu.

For more information about the Institute of Medicine, visit the IOM home page at: www.iom.edu.

The serpent has been a symbol of long life, healing, and knowledge among almost all cultures and religions since the beginning of recorded history. The serpent adopted as a logotype by the Institute of Medicine is a relief carving from ancient Greece, now held by the Staatliche Museen in Berlin.

"Knowing is not enough; we must apply. Willing is not enough; we must do."
—Goethe

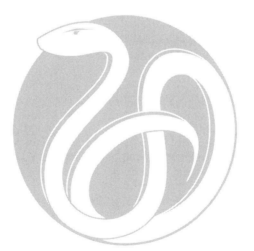

INSTITUTE OF MEDICINE
OF THE NATIONAL ACADEMIES

Advising the Nation. Improving Health.

THE NATIONAL ACADEMIES
Advisers to the Nation on Science, Engineering, and Medicine

The **National Academy of Sciences** is a private, nonprofit, self-perpetuating society of distinguished scholars engaged in scientific and engineering research, dedicated to the furtherance of science and technology and to their use for the general welfare. Upon the authority of the charter granted to it by the Congress in 1863, the Academy has a mandate that requires it to advise the federal government on scientific and technical matters. Dr. Ralph J. Cicerone is president of the National Academy of Sciences.

The **National Academy of Engineering** was established in 1964, under the charter of the National Academy of Sciences, as a parallel organization of outstanding engineers. It is autonomous in its administration and in the selection of its members, sharing with the National Academy of Sciences the responsibility for advising the federal government. The National Academy of Engineering also sponsors engineering programs aimed at meeting national needs, encourages education and research, and recognizes the superior achievements of engineers. Dr. Wm. A. Wulf is president of the National Academy of Engineering.

The **Institute of Medicine** was established in 1970 by the National Academy of Sciences to secure the services of eminent members of appropriate professions in the examination of policy matters pertaining to the health of the public. The Institute acts under the responsibility given to the National Academy of Sciences by its congressional charter to be an adviser to the federal government and, upon its own initiative, to identify issues of medical care, research, and education. Dr. Harvey V. Fineberg is president of the Institute of Medicine.

The **National Research Council** was organized by the National Academy of Sciences in 1916 to associate the broad community of science and technology with the Academy's purposes of furthering knowledge and advising the federal government. Functioning in accordance with general policies determined by the Academy, the Council has become the principal operating agency of both the National Academy of Sciences and the National Academy of Engineering in providing services to the government, the public, and the scientific and engineering communities. The Council is administered jointly by both Academies and the Institute of Medicine. Dr. Ralph J. Cicerone and Dr. Wm. A. Wulf are chair and vice chair, respectively, of the National Research Council.

www.national-academies.org

---

[2]Served through July 2006.
[3]Served through February 2006.

Reviewers

This report has been reviewed in draft form by individuals chosen for their diverse perspectives and technical expertise, in accordance with procedures approved by the National Research Council's Report Review Committee. The purpose of this independent review is to provide candid and critical comments that will assist the institution in making its published report as sound as possible and to ensure that the report meets institutional standards for objectivity, evidence, and responsiveness to the study charge. The review comments and draft manuscript remain confidential to protect the integrity of the deliberative process. We wish to thank the following individuals for their review of this report:

BRUCE BAGLEY, Medical Director for Quality Improvement, American Academy of Family Physicians, Leawood, KS

BRUCE A. BOISSONAULT, President and Chief Executive Officer, Niagara Health Quality Coalition, Williamsville, NY

TROYEN A. BRENNAN, Chief Medical Officer, Aetna, Inc., Hartford, CT

KATHLEEN BUTO, Vice President of Health Policy, Johnson and Johnson, Washington, DC

PAUL B. GINSBURG, President, Center for Studying Health System Change, Washington, DC

EMMETT KEELER, RAND Corporation, Santa Monica, CA

PETER V. LEE, President and Chief Executive Officer, Pacific Business Group on Health, San Francisco, CA

RICARDO MARTINEZ, Executive Vice President of Medical Affairs
    and Regional Medical Officer, The Schumacher Group, Decatur, GA
ARNOLD MILSTEIN, Mercer Health & Benefits, San Francisco, CA
SAM NUSSBAUM, Executive Vice President and Chief Medical
    Officer, Anthem Blue Cross Blue Shield, Indianapolis, IN
L. GREGORY PAWLSON, Executive Vice President, National
    Committee for Quality Assurance, Washington, DC
MICHAEL ROBBINS-ROTHMAN, Senior Consultant, Clinical
    Systems Improvement, University of Mississippi Medical Center,
    Jackson
VINOD K. SAHNEY, Senior Vice President and Chief Strategy
    Officer, Blue Cross Blue Shield of Massachusetts, Boston
CARY SENNETT, Senior Vice President for Research and
    Development, American Board of Internal Medicine,
    Philadelphia, PA
KENNETH E. THORPE, Robert W. Woodruff Professor and Chair
    of the Department of Health Policy and Management, Emory
    University, Rollins School of Public Health, Atlanta, GA

Although the reviewers listed above have provided many constructive comments and suggestions, they were not asked to endorse the conclusions or recommendations nor did they see the final draft of the report before its release. The review of this report was overseen by coordinator **DONALD M. STEINWACHS,** Professor and Chair, Johns Hopkins Bloomberg School of Public Health, Baltimore, MD, and monitor **HAROLD C. SOX,** Editor, *Annals of Internal Medicine*, Philadelphia, PA. Appointed by the Institute of Medicine and the National Research Council, they were responsible for making certain that an independent examination of this report was carried out in accordance with institutional procedures and that all review comments were carefully considered. Responsibility for the final content of this report rests entirely with the authoring committee and the institution.

Advisory Subcommittees

The authoring committee was assisted by three advisory subcommittees of individuals who brought additional expertise and complementary perspectives to the effort. While the groups were advisory and did not author or sign off on the reports, they did provide advice and in-depth expertise in support of their respective topics. The committee and the Institute of Medicine are grateful to them.

PAY FOR PERFORMANCE

ROBERT D. REISCHAUER (Co-Chair)*
The Urban Institute,
Washington, DC
STEPHANIE ALEXANDER
Premier, Inc., Charlotte, NC
CHARLIE D. BAKER
Harvard Pilgrim Health Care,
Wellesley, MA
JANET M. CORRIGAN*
National Quality Forum,
Washington, DC
KAREN DAVIS*
The Commonwealth Fund,
New York, NY

GAIL R. WILENSKY (Co-Chair)*
Project HOPE, Washington, DC
L. GORGON MOORE
University of Rochester, Faculty
Practice Plan, Rochester, NY
DEBRA L. NESS
National Partnership for
Women and Families,
Washington, DC
NEIL R. POWE*
Johns Hopkins University
School of Medicine and Johns
Hopkins Bloomberg School of
Public Health, Baltimore, MD

---

*Member of authorizing committee.

ARNOLD M. EPSTEIN
Harvard School of Public
Health, Boston, MA
ELLIOTT S. FISHER*
Dartmouth Medical School,
Hanover, NH
ROBERT S. GALVIN*
General Electric Company,
Fairfield, CT
SAM HO
PacifiCare Health Plans,
Cypress, CA
BARBARA B. MANARD
American Association of Homes
and Services for the Aging,
Washington, DC

CHRISTOPHER QUERAM*
Wisconsin Collaborative for
Healthcare Quality, Madison,
WI
W. ALLEN SCHAFFER
West Hartford, CT
CHERYL M. SCOTT*
Bill and Melinda Gates
Foundation, Seattle, WA
JOHN TOUSSAINT
ThedaCare, Appleton, WI

PERFORMANCE MEASUREMENT

DONALD M. BERWICK
(Co-Chair) *
Institute for Healthcare
Improvement,
Cambridge, MA
PATRICIA A. GABOW
Denver Health and Hospital
Authority,
Denver, CO
LILLEE GELINAS
VHA, Inc., Irving, TX
MARGARITA P. HURTADO
American Institutes for
Research,
Silver Spring, MD
GEORGE J. ISHAM
HealthPartners, Inc.,
Minneapolis, MN
BRENT C. JAMES
Intermountain Health Care, Salt
Lake City, UT

ELLIOTT S. FISHER
(Co-Chair) *
Dartmouth Medical School,
Hanover, NH
ELIZABETH A. MCGLYNN
RAND Corporation, Santa
Monica, CA
ARNOLD S. MILSTEIN
Mercer Health & Benefits,
San Francisco, CA
SHARON-LISE NORMAND
Harvard Medical School,
Boston, MA
BARBARA R. PAUL
Beverly Enterprises, Inc.,
Fort Smith, AR
SAMUEL O. THIER*
Harvard Medical School,
Massachusetts General Hospital,
Boston, MA

---

*Member of authorizing committee.

ARTHUR LEVIN
Center for Medical Consumers,
New York, NY
GLEN P. MAYS
University of Arkansas for
Medical Sciences,
Little Rock, AR

PAUL J. WALLACE
Kaiser Permanente Care
Management Institute,
Oakland, CA

QUALITY IMPROVEMENT ORGANIZATION
PROGRAM EVALUATION

STEPHEN M. SHORTELL
(Chair)[*]
University of California,
Berkeley
ANNE-MARIE AUDET
The Commonwealth Fund,
New York, NY
JACK L. COX
Premier, Inc., Charlotte, NC
DAVID H. GUSTAFSON[*]
University of Wisconsin,
Madison
JEFF KANG
CIGNA Health Care,
Hartford, CT
ALAN R. NELSON[*]
American College of Physicians,
Fairfax, VA

GREGG PANE
District of Columbia
Department of Health,
Washington, DC
BARBARA R. PAUL
Beverly Enterprises, Inc.,
Fort Smith, AR
WILLIAM A. PECK[*]
Washington University School
of Medicine,
St. Louis, MO
ERIC D. PETERSON
Duke University School of
Medicine, Durham, NC
SHOSHANNA SOFAER
Baruch College, New York, NY

---

[*]Member of authorizing committee.

Foreword

This report is the third in a series called *Pathways to Quality Health Care*. Led by the Committee on Redesigning Health Insurance Performance Measures, Payment, and Performance Improvement Programs, these reports promote a health system that meets patients' needs and is based on sound scientific evidence. The *Pathways* series extends the work inaugurated by the Institute of Medicine (IOM) in its 2001 report *Crossing the Quality Chasm*. That earlier report laid out a blueprint for reforming health care through systems improvement. The new series of reports provides strategies for creating and implementing change that will help bridge the quality chasm.

The Committee on Redesigning Health Insurance Performance Measures, Payment, and Performance Improvement Programs was composed of 23 individuals who are among the top experts and leaders on health care in the country. They and IOM staff carefully reviewed the literature and gathered data on measurement, quality improvement, and pay for performance to provide an evidence base for the *Pathways* reports. Although the committee members come from different backgrounds, disciplines, and perspectives, they reached a common understanding of the problems to be addressed, shared a sense of urgency, and converged on three major sets of recommendations. The committee saw the need to reform health care payment methods that promote inappropriate or inefficient behaviors and that impede progress toward better quality care. Their central ideas about payment that rewards higher quality, establishment of a National Quality Coordination Board to guide performance measurement, and restructuring

Quality Improvement Organizations to offer technical assistance in the best methods to increase quality all point to a better-performing health system.

Requests for this report, as well as the preceding two in the *Pathways* series, were embedded in the Medicare Modernization Act, and therefore focus on Medicare programs. The committee's recommendations, like the Medicare program itself, ramify beyond Medicare's direct beneficiaries. Implementation of these recommendations by the Medicare program could influence adoption by other purchasers and payers of care. Medicare's use of particular performance standards can eventually raise the quality of care all Americans receive.

Chairman Steven A. Schroeder has skillfully guided this committee through three important studies. He and all of the committee members deserve our thanks for so generously contributing their time and expertise. They served as volunteers for more than 2 years, and their individual and collective commitment to improving the quality of health care is laudable. By implementing their recommendations, we can convert their service into results that benefit all Americans.

Harvey V. Fineberg, M.D., Ph.D.
President, Institute of Medicine
August 2006

Preface

Rewarding Provider Performance: Aligning Incentives in Medicare is the third and final report of the Committee on Redesigning Health Insurance Performance Measures, Payment, and Performance Improvement Programs. This committee's efforts have been in response to two separate congressional mandates embodied in the Medicare Prescription Drug, Improvement, and Modernization Act of 2003 (Public Law 108-173, Sections 109 and 238). These mandates provided the Institute of Medicine with the opportunity to build on an earlier series of reports, called the *Quality Chasm* series, which created a goal for the American health system of health care that is safe, effective, patient-centered, timely, efficient, and equitable. This committee's three reports form a new series, called *Pathways to Quality Health Care*, which offers strategies for achieving that goal.

The first report in the *Pathways* series, *Performance Measurement: Accelerating Improvement*, focused on measuring the quality of health care services. Many individuals and organizations, as well as health care providers, are working on creating, implementing, and reporting measures to determine how well health care is delivered. The committee perceived a national need to standardize measures in order to minimize the burden on providers of collecting and reporting data and to facilitate the use of this information by consumers and purchasers of services. Thus, it recommended a starter set of performance measures and areas in which measures need to be developed. To coordinate the implementation of a standard set of performance measures, further the research and development needed to create and implement new measures, and facilitate public reporting, the committee recommended a National Quality Coordination Board.

In its second report, *Medicare's Quality Improvement Organization Program: Maximizing Potential*, the committee examined the Quality Improvement Organization (QIO) program in Medicare. It concluded that the QIO program could form a critical infrastructure to help improve providers' performance and their reporting of measures. Given the growing emphasis on performance measurement and public reporting of those measures for a broad range of health care providers, as well as payment incentives, the committee expects providers to increasingly seek assistance from their local QIO. The committee recommended that the program be restructured to focus on technical assistance to health care providers and to strengthen the governance of QIOs and program management.

For this third report, the committee examined the evidence concerning various public- and private-sector programs designed to align payment incentives to promote better-quality care by rewarding providers who perform well. Because the current basic payment systems reward overuse of services and use of high-cost complex procedures and do not acknowledge the wide variations in quality across providers, the committee concluded that payment reforms are needed now to recognize care that is of high clinical quality, patient-centered, and efficient. To help implement payment incentives within Medicare, the committee proposes a phased approach and offers guidance on creating pools of funds to reward performance and submission of performance data, and mechanisms for monitoring of implementation to avoid unintended consequences. The committee believes that implementation of the recommendations in all three reports would provide a strong start toward improving the quality of care for all Americans.

It has been an honor to serve as chair of the Committee on Redesigning Health Insurance Performance Measures, Payment, and Performance Improvement Programs, and I am grateful to all the committee members and staff for their hard work, willingness to reach consensus, and ability to produce such an ambitious series of reports. I especially want to recognize the members of the Subcommittee on Pay for Performance and its co-chairs, Robert Reischauer and Gail Wilensky, for their contributions to this report. Also, Rosemary Chalk deserves particular thanks for taking over as project director. Our collective efforts have produced these three reports; it is now up to you, our readers, and your various communities, along with Congress and the Centers for Medicare and Medicaid Services, to make the vision contained in these reports a reality.

Steven A. Schroeder, M.D.
Chairman
August 2006

Acknowledgments

Rewarding Provider Performance: Aligning Incentives in Medicare benefited from the contributions of many individuals. The committee takes this opportunity to recognize those who so generously gave their time and expertise to inform its deliberations. The committee wishes to acknowledge the members of the Subcommittee on Pay for Performance and the outstanding leadership of co-chairs Robert Reischauer (Urban Institute) and Gail Wilensky (Project HOPE). John Ring and Clyde Behney also contributed as directors of the Board on Health Care Services of the Institute of Medicine.

The committee benefited from presentations made by a number of experts. The following individuals shared their experiences and perspectives: Trent Haywood and Lisa Magno from the Centers for Medicare and Medicaid Services (CMS) on CMS's pay-for-performance initiatives; Francois deBrantes from Bridges to Excellence (BTE) on incentivizing patients/consumers and lessons learned from the development of the BTE program; Bruce Landon and Meredith Rosenthal through their commissioned paper "Paying for Physician Quality in Traditional Medicare"; Mark Miller and Karen Milgate of the Medicare Payment Advisory Commission (MedPAC), on MedPAC's recommendations on pay for performance and also Medicare data runs; and Shari Erickson of the National Quality Forum on health information technology. We would also like to thank those representatives of the various medical associations who generously provided presentations addressing their organizations' positions on pay for performance, including Nancy Nielson of the American Medical Association, John Tooker of the American College of Physicians, Rosemarie Sweeney of the American Academy of Family Physicians, Carole Johnson of the Alliance of Community Health Plans, Frederick L. Grover and Jeffrey Rich of the Society of Thoracic Surgeons, Joseph S. Bailes of the American Society of Clinical Oncology, William L. Rich III of the American Academy of Ophthalmology, and Arl Van Moore Jr. of the American College of Radiology.

The committee would like to acknowledge organizations that provided us with feedback on their pay-for-performance position statements: Alliance of Community Health Plans, Alliance of Specialty Medicine, American Academy of Family Physicians, American College of Cardiology, American College of Physicians, American Medical Association, National Business Group on Health, National Patient Advocacy Foundation, and Society of Thoracic Surgeons.

We also wish to acknowledge Marie-Adele Sorel, a Truman Scholar during the summer of 2005, who provided significant contributions to this report. Thanks to Meredith Rosenthal for consulting on this report.

Finally, the committee gratefully acknowledges CMS, whose funding supported this congressionally mandated study.

Contents

REWARDING PROVIDER
PERFORMANCE

Summary

The overall quality of health care delivered to Americans is worse than it should be. While many quality improvement efforts have been undertaken, their success has been limited by current payment systems. The existing systems do not reflect the relative value of health care services in important aspects of quality, such as clinical quality, patient-centeredness, and efficiency. Nor do current payment systems recognize or reward care coordination, an omission reflected in such shortcomings as the limited focus on prevention and the treatment of chronic conditions as patients move across various care settings. Fundamental changes in approaches to health care payment are necessary to remove impediments to and create incentives for significant quality improvement.

The Institute of Medicine (IOM) report *Crossing the Quality Chasm: A New Health System for the 21st Century* made the case for changes in the health care system, including restructuring of payment methods, to close the quality gap. Five years later, however, the concerns raised in that report persist. The report identified six aims for health care that should guide quality improvement efforts—safety, effectiveness, patient-centeredness, timeliness, efficiency, and equity—and noted that payment systems supporting the organization and delivery of the nation's health care services do not align incentives to support the realization of these aims. Instead, current payment policies reinforce the existing organizational structure and delivery processes of the American health care system by paying according to the number and complexity of services by setting rather than recognizing the relative value of those services. New payment incentives must be created to encourage the redesign of structures and processes of care to promote higher value. Although the magnitude of incentives necessary to achieve significant and sustainable change while avoiding adverse consequences is uncertain, steps can be taken now to begin to address the deficiencies of current payment systems and encourage progress toward significant quality improvement.

STUDY CHARGE AND SCOPE

This study is the third in the IOM's *Pathways to Quality Health Care* series, which offers tools for implementing the vision of improved health care delineated in the *Quality Chasm* report. The first report in the *Pathways* series, *Performance Measurement: Accelerating Improvement*, recommended a strategy for developing and implementing a comprehensive performance measurement system, including creation of a national board to coordinate that effort. The second report, *Medicare's Quality Improvement Organization Program: Maximizing Potential*, recommended an emphasis on technical assistance to providers for quality improvement. The present report builds on those studies and offers an operational plan for introducing into Medicare payment incentives that would encourage and reward high-quality care. While alignment can occur in many areas, this report is limited to examining the link between payment incentives and provider performance.

In the context of current efforts to test pay for performance in both the public and private sectors, the U.S. Congress, as part of the Medicare Prescription Drug, Improvement, and Modernization Act of 2003 (Public Law 108-173, Section 238), directed the IOM to identify and prioritize options for aligning performance with payment in the Medicare program under Title XVIII of the Social Security Act (42 U.S.C. 1395 et seq.). The congressional mandate identified three topics for the study to address:

- The performance measure set to be used and how that set should be updated.
- The payment policy that should be used to reward performance.
- The key implementation issues involved, such as data and information technology requirements.

In response to this mandate, the IOM Committee on Redesigning Health Insurance Performance Measures, Payment, and Performance Improvement Programs explored the design and implementation of payment rewards for performance in Medicare. It considered both specific topics involved in introducing pay for performance within Medicare and the implications of using this payment approach as part of a long-term multipayer effort to better align the health care system with a vision of quality.

PAY FOR PERFORMANCE: AN IMMEDIATE OPPORTUNITY

The objective of aligning incentives through pay for performance—paying providers for higher-quality care as measured by selected standards and procedures—is to create payment incentives that will:

- Encourage the most rapid feasible performance improvement by all providers.
- Support innovation and constructive change throughout the health care system.
- Promote better outcomes of care, especially through coordination of care across provider settings and time.

Pay for performance is not simply a mechanism to reward those who perform well or to reduce costs. Its purpose is to align payment incentives to encourage ongoing improvement in a way that will ensure high-quality care for all. Pay for performance will not necessarily reduce the cost of care, but it will help ensure that what is paid for will be more beneficial to patients. In theory, payment incentives induce certain predictable responses or behaviors. The notion that paying more for some attribute of a good or service will stimulate further production of that attribute is fundamental in most sectors of the economy, but the explicit linkage of incentives to quality and performance in health care markets is a relatively new concept. Therefore, introducing payment incentives to reward high quality in a national health care program requires attention to effects on providers, purchasers, health plans, and consumers.

More than 100 reward and incentive payment programs have been launched in the private health care sector. Most of these efforts have not yet been fully evaluated. The Centers for Medicare and Medicaid Services (CMS) in the U.S. Department of Health and Human Services (DHHS) has also initiated a series of demonstration projects to explore the potential of pay for performance to achieve quality improvement in Medicare. Some of these programs have begun to show that providers respond positively to payment incentives that promote and reward quality improvement practices, but it remains unknown whether the improvements seen will be significant and sustained. The literature evaluating the effectiveness of pay for performance consists of fewer than 20 studies, yielding mixed conclusions on overall impact. Some studies have shown a positive effect on the quality of care, but others have not demonstrated this relationship. In general, the effect of most of these programs has not been examined sufficiently. Despite these uncertainties, however, Medicare payment systems, if left unchanged, will pose a barrier to improved health care quality.

MEDICARE AND PAYMENT INCENTIVES

Medicare, the government health program for the elderly (ages 65 and over) and qualified disabled populations, covered nearly 42 million Americans in 2004. Medicare is the nation's largest single payer for health care services, with total expenditures of $309 billion in 2004, and this amount is estimated to grow rapidly. Although Medicare is federally administered and largely federally financed, its beneficiaries are served almost entirely by private providers. For services provided to the 88 percent (approximately 37 million) of beneficiaries enrolled in the traditional fee-for-service option, Medicare pays providers amounts that are set prospectively on the basis of resource cost and complexity of services delivered. For the remaining 12 percent of beneficiaries who have opted to receive their Medicare services from private plans participating in the Medicare Advantage program, Medicare pays a fixed, risk-adjusted monthly amount per beneficiary to the plans, which in turn pay providers via diverse methods.

The current Medicare fee-for-service payment system is unlikely to promote quality improvement because it tends to reward excessive use of services; high-cost, complex procedures; and lower-quality care. Through bundled and prospective payment arrangements for institutions, Medicare has attempted to create incentives for efficiencies, but significant price and payment distortions persist.

Services that contribute greatly to high-quality care that are labor- or time-intensive and rely less on technical resources, such as patient education in self-management of chronic conditions and care coordination, tend to be undervalued and are not adequately reflected in current payment arrangements. Little emphasis is placed on efficiency (achieving high clinical quality with a given amount of resources). The lack of incentives for comprehensive, coordinated care discourages services targeting early intervention and prevention that can ultimately reduce the use of expensive services, such as avoidable hospitalizations. Providers often miss opportunities for collaboration since the payment system rewards neither team management nor the integration of services across care settings. Medicare's fee-for-service payments, the relative profitability per service, and most private purchasers' payment mechanisms create incentives for providers to specialize in fields that are more resource-intensive at the expense of primary care, which has not fared well under the current Medicare reimbursement systems.

Aligning payment incentives with quality improvement goals represents a promising opportunity to encourage higher levels of quality and provide better value for all Americans. However, pay for performance needs to be closely monitored because it could have unintended adverse consequences, such as decreased access to care, increased disparities in care, or impediments to innovation. Careful monitoring of implementation should minimize any such adverse consequences. The committee thus reached two key conclusions regarding pay for performance as a new payment strategy for Medicare:

> The systematic and deliberate use of payment incentives that recognize and reward high levels of quality and quality improvement can serve as a powerful stimulus to drive institutional and provider behavior toward better quality.
>
> The incentives introduced by pay for performance, by themselves, will not be sufficient to achieve the broad institutional and behavioral changes needed unless certain operating conditions are met, such as the use of electronic health records, public reporting, beneficiary incentives, and education of boards of directors, which could lead to significant and synergistic gains in quality improvement.

INITIAL IMPLEMENTATION: A PHASED APPROACH

While an evidence base is not yet available for determining with certainty what type of payment incentive strategy would best advance the quality improvement agenda, experiences with pay for performance to date have been promising. Consequently, the committee favors an approach that would capture key lessons from these early experiences and maintain the flexibility to make subsequent changes where necessary. Specifically, the committee concludes pay for performance should be introduced through a phased approach: rewarding performance in selected settings, with a small level of funding, on specific measures, and moving eventually to include all provider settings, with a larger level of funding, on more measures. Such a phased approach requires attention to the timing and pace of implementation for specific settings, reward amounts, and measures. A phased approach also provides an opportunity to examine other long-term approaches.

Pay for performance in Medicare can help address current problems and stimulate complementary quality improvement strategies. Indeed, the long-term potential of pay for performance may lie in its ability to encourage the use of mutually reinforcing quality improvement strategies, such as technical assistance, use of information technology, professional certification, public reporting, and provider and consumer education. Pay for performance cannot significantly improve quality and reduce costs in isolation from other changes in the Medicare system, and could in fact pose a barrier to achieving the transformational changes required to improve care if implemented in ways that would reinforce the current fragmented delivery system. The hope is that payment incentives can offer a stimulus to move health care practices overall from the status quo toward new organizational and individual behaviors that will result in better quality of care.

Recommendation 1: The Secretary of the Department of Health and Human Services (DHHS) should implement pay for performance in Medicare using a phased approach as a stimulus to foster comprehensive and systemwide improvements in the quality of health care.

Achieving the promise of pay for performance to recognize and reward quality in Medicare requires answer to questions about several key design features, including:

- The sources of revenue for rewards.
- The types of performance measures that should receive preferential treatment in the early stages of implementation.
- The appropriate design of the reward system.

The performance measurement framework will have to be sophisticated and nuanced to account fairly for complex clinical situations, such as the treatment of patients with multiple chronic diseases, in which the accepted care for one condition may be in conflict with that for another. Complex measures to address concerns about efficiency and patient-centeredness will require attention. Providers in different institutional settings (e.g., hospitals or skilled nursing facilities), diverse organizational environments (e.g., managed care or solo practices), and different specialty fields will need new capabilities (e.g., databases, information tools, and technical assistance) to comply with new reporting and payment procedures. If payment incentives are not carefully aligned with desired outcomes or if adequate resources or risk adjustments are not readily available, some providers may avoid accepting patients whose conditions could jeopardize their performance rating.

Recognizing the complexities of current circumstances, as well as the demand for action, the committee emphasizes the importance of introducing pay for performance not only through a gradual and phased approach that varies by setting, amount of reward, and measure, but also within a learning system that can evaluate experience with early efforts. Caution must be exercised to ensure that the proposed phased approach does not widen current gaps in performance among providers and domains of care. A learning system depends on monitoring and evaluation and collaboration between the private and public sectors that enables all stakeholders to learn from experience. Ultimately, major restructuring of basic Medicare payment systems beyond the incentives discussed in this report will be necessary. Such restructuring, which could require a transformation away from fee-for-service payments, could include elevating the value of integrated care management, relying more heavily on electronic health records, and facilitating payment that rewards high performance and coordination of services across care settings. Because measures and information systems needed to monitor both meaningful outcomes of care and the health status of patients across different care settings are not yet available, this shift would have to occur in the future. Further research will be necessary to develop benchmarks that can guide the process of phased implementation and restructuring of payment arrangements.

FUNDING OF PAY FOR PERFORMANCE

There are three potential sources of funding for a pay-for-performance program in Medicare: (1) existing funds, (2) generated savings, and (3) new money. Combinations of these sources are used in current pay-for-performance experiments, though new money is rarely agreeable to payers. Existing funds represent monies that are already projected to be part of the payment system. Payment incentives could be financed by reducing the base payments of all providers or by reducing scheduled payment increases. These funds would then be awarded to high-quality providers. Alternatively, a portion of each payment could be withheld, with the balance returned to those providers who achieved quality goals. However, rewards would initially be small; for example, modeling reductions in all payments by 2 percent for three clinical conditions resulted in physician rewards averaging $88 per physician per year (assuming that half of treating physicians would qualify for rewards). The generated-savings model creates a reward pool through cost-reducing reforms and efficiencies; however, these efficiencies have not yet been adequately demonstrated in pay-for-performance efforts. The new-money model taps the Medicare Trust Funds or calls for a separate appropriation of general revenues that would be awarded as bonuses to high-quality providers in addition to the scheduled base payments and updates all providers receive.

The committee used four criteria to assess the appropriateness of these three possible funding sources: adequacy, stability, fairness, and impact. In addition, the committee gave overall priority to funding approaches that would be budget conscious (or, preferably, budget neutral), ensuring that budget concerns would be explicitly recognized and addressed.

Recommendation 2: Congress should derive initial funding (over the next 3–5 years) for a pay-for-performance program in Medicare largely from existing funds.

- **Congress should create provider-specific pools from a reduction in the base Medicare payments for each class of providers (hospitals, skilled nursing facilities, Medicare Advantage plans, dialysis facilities, home health agencies, and physicians).**

- Congress should ensure that these pools are large enough to create adequate motivation for improved performance on selected measures. Because of unique challenges of physician payment relating to the sustainable growth rate (SGR), investment dollars may be necessary to create adequate resources to effect change.
- Initial funding should be budget conscious in taking into account the resources needed for both funding the pools and implementing the program.

Because the proposed pools would be created by reducing base payments for all Medicare providers in each setting, all should have the opportunity to participate in the performance reward program. New money may initially be necessary in some provider settings to create adequate resources to influence change. The feasibility of using other funding sources, particularly the generated-savings model, should be tested and evaluated over the next 3–5 years to assess the likely impacts and consequences.

One of the primary goals of new payment incentives should be to stimulate collaboration and shared accountability among providers across care settings for better patient-centered health outcomes. Although the implementation of pay for performance will most likely begin with pools created by setting, CMS should build toward an ultimate vision of aggregating funds for rewards into one integrated pool that would accommodate shared accountability and encourage coordination of care.

> **Recommendation 3: Congress should give the Secretary of DHHS the authority to aggregate the pools for different care settings into one consolidated pool from which all providers would be rewarded when the development of new performance measures allows for shared accountability and more coordinated care across provider settings.**

STRUCTURE OF REWARDS

CMS will have many issues to consider in the distribution of rewards, such as what measures to use in assessing performance and how performance should translate into rewards for individual providers. The magnitude and relative distribution of rewards should depend on program priorities; little evidence exists to guide the distribution of rewards. Continuous monitoring and adjustment will be necessary to ensure that providers are appropriately rewarded for the care they deliver. In the absence of evidence, the committee provides recommendations in two key areas: rewards for specific domains of quality and performance objectives.

Rewards for Specific Domains of Quality

The ultimate goal of pay for performance is to improve quality and patient outcomes. However, current capabilities focus largely on measuring processes of care. Many providers are skeptical that reliable and valid performance measures can be introduced for complex clinical processes. They are also doubtful that incentives can be instituted to reward performance in areas that truly matter—those necessary to improve the health and care of their patients. A major challenge confronting the introduction of pay for performance, therefore, is overcoming the fear that efforts to improve upon one domain of performance may lead to reductions in quality in other domains. Under a new payment mechanism, for example, improved efficiency may greatly benefit the overall quality of the system, yet more important, it may also compromise clinical quality or patient-centered care. Similarly, many purchasers and public officials are concerned that focusing on enhancing clinical quality or patient-centered care will not adequately address concerns about the growing costs of health services or reduce current waste and inefficiencies.

To create new payment incentives that can foster overall quality improvement and better patient outcomes, the committee consolidated the six quality aims of the *Quality Chasm* report into three domains—clinical quality, patient-centered care, and efficiency. Eventually, if pay for performance is found to have positive effects, other aspects of care should also be measured and rewarded.

Recommendation 4: In designing a pay-for-performance program, the Secretary of DHHS should initially reward health care that is of high clinical quality, patient-centered, and efficient.

Performance Objectives

Two categories of performance benchmarks deserve consideration in designing a payment incentive program: (1) improvement—rewarding all providers who demonstrate significant improvement, and (2) excellence—rewarding those providers who meet or exceed a recognized threshold of desired quality. Current private-sector pay-for-performance programs have reward structures that utilize one or both of these categories.

Recommendation 5: The Secretary of DHHS should design a pay-for-performance program that initially rewards both providers who improve performance significantly and those who achieve high performance.

The distribution of rewards for both improvement and excellence would allow providers at all performance levels to find at least one of these goals within reach. The fraction of rewards allocated to improve on a given measure set should be reduced over time to only reward care that is truly of high performance. As providers make significant improvements on basic measures, the allocation of rewards for those measures should shift in favor of higher payments for more complex indices of performance. Rewards should also shift to reflect progress in the development of new measure sets and changes in priorities. Even when measure sets or priorities are stable, the focus of rewards should be altered to ensure that providers do not focus their performance improvement efforts too narrowly.

IMPLEMENTATION

CMS will also need to address procedural and technical issues, including the following:

- The procedures by which comparative information on provider performance will be released to the public.
- Ways of overcoming the barriers to participation.
- The process of improving care coordination among providers serving the same patient.
- The role of information technology use in supporting better care delivery and a performance-based payment strategy.

Public Reporting and Transparency

Beyond merely collecting data on provider performance, CMS should make such data publicly available so that consumers will have the opportunity to fully characterize the performance of providers when making health care decisions. Public disclosure of information, with necessary patient protections, can also stimulate higher levels of quality by showing providers how their performance compares with that of their peers. While the evidence remains mixed, peer comparisons may be a more powerful force than monetary incentives in encouraging providers to adopt practices that improve quality of care. However, payment incentives are necessary as a key stimulus to foster widespread public reporting.

Recommendation 6: Because public reporting of performance measures should be an integral component of a pay-for-performance program for Medicare, the Secretary of DHHS should offer incentives to providers for the submission of performance data, and ensure that information pertaining to provider performance is

transparent and made public in ways that are both meaningful and understandable to consumers.

The committee proposes that public reporting requirements precede changes in payment strategies to allow time for providers to give feedback on performance results and comparisons. To advance the pace of adoption, incentives should be offered for the submission of performance measurement data that contributes to public reports. Public reports can inform consumer choices only if they are presented in a manner that is meaningful and easily understandable. Over time, payment incentives for the submission of routine data should be phased out so that this pool of funds can be redirected to the development of measures for areas that are more difficult to assess.

Ways of Overcoming Barriers to Participation

In its deliberations, the committee recognized the importance of establishing the expectation that all Medicare providers would participate in public reporting and pay for performance. However, it also recognized that the pace of implementation, the breadth of measure sets applicable to specific types of providers, and the size and distribution of reward pools would need to vary depending on the availability of measures and the organizational and technological challenges faced by different providers in carrying out performance measurement and reporting.

Many types of Medicare providers, including hospitals, home health agencies, and Medicare Advantage plans, are already submitting performance data for public reporting. For these providers, CMS should begin pay-for-performance programs on existing measures immediately, and move toward comprehensive performance assessment systems and sizable reward pools during the next 3 years.

Although skilled nursing facilities are already publicly reporting data to CMS, the performance measures reflecting their treatment of Medicare beneficiaries are not yet adequate to support pay for performance. There are also currently few, if any, performance measures for other providers, such as clinical laboratories and ambulatory surgical centers. Efforts should begin immediately to develop and test performance measure sets so that these providers can begin to participate in public reporting and pay for performance as soon as possible.

CMS has already begun a voluntary reporting program for physicians on selected measures. CMS should immediately develop and implement a strategy for ensuring that virtually all physicians participate—on at least some measures—as soon as possible. This strategy will need to be sensitive to differences across specialties in the availability of performance measures and the diversity of information systems and operational supports in various practice settings. Financial incentives adequate to ensure early and broad physician participation in the submission of performance measures and public reporting should be used. Consideration should be given to benefits such as linking accelerated payments or the physician annual payment update to public reporting. Initial measure sets for pay for performance may need to be limited in some physician settings. In establishing the size of the reward pools proposed above, CMS will need to strike a balance between providing financial incentives sizable enough to lead to near-universal participation and recognizing that initial measure sets are narrow, presenting an incomplete picture of a provider's performance.

The transformational changes in the health care delivery system envisioned in the *Pathways* series of reports will depend upon the adoption of both longitudinal measures of quality that cut across settings and payment rewards that are substantial. The pay-for-performance strategy should move as soon as practical from a relatively narrow, provider-specific approach to a more comprehensive, longitudinal set of measures and substantial rewards that encompass all Medicare providers.

A monitoring system should be incorporated into the implementation process to inform future decisions about the pace of expansion of performance measure sets and make it possible to determine whether the voluntary approach initially recommended for physicians is achieving the goal of near-universal participation.

Recommendation 7: The Secretary of DHHS should develop and implement a strategy for ensuring that virtually all Medicare providers submit performance measures for public reporting and participate in pay for performance as soon as possible. Initially, measure sets may need to be narrow, but they should evolve over time to provide more comprehensive and longitudinal assessments of provider and system performance. For many institutional providers, participation in public reporting and pay for performance can and should begin immediately. For physicians, a voluntary approach should be pursued initially, relying on financial incentives sufficient to ensure broad participation and recognizing that the initial set of measures and the pace of expansion of measure sets will need to be sensitive to the operational challenges faced by providers in small practice settings. Three years after the release of this report, the Secretary of DHHS should determine whether progress toward universal participation is sufficient and whether stronger actions—such as mandating provider participation—are required.

Care Coordination

Rewarding providers on the basis of performance will require that Medicare know which providers delivered care to specific patients. Patients frequently interact with more than one provider, and treatment of complex conditions often requires consultation with multiple specialists. On average, Medicare beneficiaries are treated annually by 5 physicians; beneficiaries with the chronic conditions of chronic heart failure, coronary artery disease, and diabetes see an average of 13 physicians annually. Enhancing care coordination is essential to improving quality.

> **Recommendation 8: The Centers for Medicare and Medicaid Services (CMS) should design the Medicare pay-for-performance program to include components that promote, recognize, and reward improved coordination of care across providers and through entire episodes of illness. Thus, CMS should (1) encourage beneficiaries and providers to identify providers who would be considered their principal responsible source of care, and (2) pay for and reward successful care coordination that meets specified standards for providers who take on that role.**

Not all providers treating Medicare beneficiaries would be willing or able to provide this coordinating function; thus CMS should design a strategy to reward those who are capable of and willing to assume this role. Beneficiaries should be encouraged to designate their responsible sources of care through incentives such as reductions in their Medicare Part B premiums. All such activities should protect patient confidentiality and be carried out in compliance with regulations of the Health Insurance Portability and Accountability Act.

Information Technology

Information technology has enormous potential to be used as a transformative tool in systems change toward improving the quality of health care. Pay for performance can influence the rate of information technology adoption, but information technologies are not a necessary component of pay for performance. While promising, the infrastructure required to automate patient-specific clinical information has not yet fully been embraced. Without clear standards, experimentation will likely continue slowly, in a piecemeal fashion.

Recommendation 9: Because electronic health information technology will increase the probability of a successful pay-for-performance program, the Secretary of DHHS should explore a variety of approaches for assisting providers in the implementation of electronic data collection and reporting systems to strengthen the use of consistent performance measures.

MONITORING, EVALUATION, AND RESEARCH

Monitoring, evaluation, and research should be integral components of any pay-for-performance program. Issues to be addressed include use of current data to evaluate impact; processes for developing robust performance measures; and development of real-time monitoring systems to identify unintended adverse consequences. A successful pay-for-performance program must also encompass the elements of a true learning system, including having strong leadership, a shared vision, and an environment that allows for action in response to observations.

Recommendation 10: The Secretary of DHHS should implement a monitoring and evaluation system for the Medicare pay-for-performance program in order to:

- Assess early experiences with implementation so timely corrective action can be taken.
- Evaluate the overall impact of pay for performance on clinical quality, patient-centeredness, and efficiency.
- Identify the best practices of high-performing delivery settings that should be shared with others to improve care throughout the nation.

This active learning system should be complemented by a research agenda identified through consensus among the major stakeholders to create the context for future investigations as actual experience raises new questions. Research should also be aimed at building an evidence base to guide the design of future pay-for-performance programs.

Collaboration between the public and private efforts is critical. While multiple stakeholder groups are now developing reliable, valid, and accurate performance metrics in the area of clinical quality, these efforts are not coordinated and often produce competing and inconsistent measures that are burdensome to providers.

CMS should conduct demonstration projects to evaluate different options that are theoretically sound but untested. Such projects could limit risks and accelerate progress in payment realignment by confirming benefits and minimizing the risk of undue hardship for beneficiaries or providers.

1

Introduction

Health care quality in the United States falls short of its potential. Patients do not always receive the care that is best suited to their needs, and increased spending for health services does not always result in higher-quality care or better patient outcomes (IOM, 2000; Fisher et al., 2004). In some cases, the care provided can in fact be harmful; services that are not necessary, safe, or timely can put the lives and well-being of patients at risk. As a result, not only the quality but also the overall value of health care services has become questionable. In two seminal reports—*To Err Is Human: Building a Safer Health System* and *Crossing the Quality Chasm: A New Health System for the 21st Century*—the Institute of Medicine (IOM) recognized these disquieting realities and called for a restructuring of the health care system (IOM, 2000, 2001).

The *Quality Chasm* report identified ten rules for redesigning health care processes to improve performance (see Box 1-1). The report also recommended the alignment of public and private payment methods to build incentives for quality enhancement. In response to the *Quality Chasm* report, numerous reform efforts were undertaken with the goal of improving the quality of care. These efforts yielded modest gains in some areas, but have not resulted in the fundamental improvements Americans deserve. In the 5 years since the report was published, the quality of health care has remained poorer than it should be (Leape and Berwick, 2005). Transformational changes throughout the health care system are essential to close the quality gap, and these needed changes include the restructuring of payment methods.

**BOX 1-1   Ten Rules for Redesigning
Health Care Processes**

1. *Care based on continuous healing relationships.* Patients should receive care whenever they need it and in many forms, not just face-to-face visits. This rule implies that the health care system should be responsive at all times (24 hours a day, every day) and that access to care should be provided over the Internet, by telephone, and by other means in addition to face-to-face visits.

2. *Customization based on patient needs and values.* The system of care should be designed to meet the most common types of needs, but have the capability to respond to individual patient choices and preferences.

3. *The patient as the source of control.* Patients should be given the necessary information and the opportunity to exercise the degree of control they choose over health care decisions that affect them. The health system should be able to accommodate differences in patient preferences and encourage shared decision making.

4. *Shared knowledge and the free flow of information.* Patients should have unfettered access to their own medical information and to clinical knowledge. Clinicians and patients should communicate effectively and share information.

5. *Evidence-based decision making.* Patients should receive care based on the best available scientific knowledge. Care should not vary illogically from clinician to clinician or from place to place.

6. *Safety as a system property.* Patients should be safe from injury caused by the care system. Reducing risk and ensuring safety require greater attention to systems that help prevent and mitigate errors.

7. *The need for transparency.* The health care system should make information available to patients and their families that allows them to make informed decisions when selecting a health plan, hospital, or clinical practice, or choosing among alternative treatments. This should include information describing the system's performance on safety, evidence-based practice, and patient satisfaction.

8. *Anticipation of needs.* The health system should anticipate patient needs, rather than simply reacting to events.

9. *Continuous decrease in waste.* The health system should not waste resources or patient time.

10. *Cooperation among clinicians.* Clinicians and institutions should actively collaborate and communicate to ensure an appropriate exchange of information and coordination of care.

SOURCE: IOM, 2001:8–9.

STUDY CHARGE AND SCOPE

A unique opportunity to examine the contribution of and experience with pay-for-performance strategies was provided by the Medicare Prescription Drug, Improvement, and Modernization Act of 2003 (Public Law 108-173, Section 238). In this legislation, the U.S. Congress asked the IOM to conduct a study that would identify and prioritize options for aligning performance with payment in the Medicare program under Title XVIII of the Social Security Act (42 U.S.C. 1395 et seq.). The congressional mandate identified three topics for the IOM study to address:

• The performance measure set to be used and how that measure set should be updated.
• The payment policy that should be used to reward performance.
• The key implementation issues involved, such as data and information technology requirements.

In response to this mandate, the IOM charged the Committee on Redesigning Health Insurance Performance Measures, Payment, and Performance Improvement Programs to explore the implementation of rewards for provider performance in Medicare. In carrying out its charge, the committee considered the role of payment strategies within a broader set of interdependent performance improvement efforts that include performance measures, public reports, use of innovative technologies, technical assistance, provider and consumer education, provider certification processes, and new organizational structures; these efforts may all be tied to financial incentives. Taken together, these performance improvement strategies have the potential to transform the quality of health care services and the settings in which they are delivered so that greater attention is focused on what truly matters—better health and outcomes.

The committee has authored three reports, known collectively as the *Pathways to Quality Health Care* series, which explore how selected tools for improving health care quality and performance can be used to achieve better health and better value.

The first report in the *Pathways* series—*Performance Measurement: Accelerating Improvement* (IOM, 2006b)—reviewed leading health care performance measures and examined their utility in supporting quality improvement, public information, and pay-for-performance policies. The committee recommended a starter set of performance measures to stimulate data collection, reporting, and, ultimately, payment that is directed toward fostering quality improvement. This study also provided a roadmap for defining and developing measures that could capture other dimensions of quality essential to assessing the overall performance of individual providers, as well as complex organizational settings. The dimensions largely missing from currently available measures include longitudinal, population-based measures that foster shared accountability of providers. Measures emerging in these areas could yield a deeper understanding of the ways in which certain processes and relationships are linked to better health outcomes; patient experiences of care; and more efficient use of financial, human, and organizational resources. Recognizing performance measures as essential building blocks for an improved health care system, this study also recommended the formation of a new governmental entity, the National Quality Coordination Board, to offer leadership in and help standardize and coordinate performance measurement efforts.

Introducing new data collection, reporting, and payment systems throughout the health care system will require intensive collaboration, technical assistance, and information technologies that can contribute to quality improvement. Many of these issues were addressed in the second *Pathways* report, *Medicare's Quality Improvement Organization Program: Maximizing Potential* (IOM, 2006a). For example, providers need to learn more about how to improve clinical and preventive care by sharing best practices and lessons learned in the adoption of new technologies, procedures, and behavioral interventions. Technical assistance for quality improvement will become increasingly important throughout Medicare as pressure to contain health care costs grows, and providers place more emphasis on quality improvement with the expansion of pay-for-performance programs. The Quality Improvement Organization program, administered by Medicare through a series of state-based contracts, constitutes an important national resource in building the necessary infrastructure for this technical assistance. The program's goals and mission need to be redefined, however, so its efforts can focus on giving all providers the technical assistance they need to build their capacity for performance measurement and quality improvement.

In this third report in the *Pathways* series, the IOM committee builds on its earlier analyses of performance measures and quality improvement. The report specifically addresses the creation of incentives designed to reward health care providers for improvements in care, as well as for their efforts that increase the value of health care services. This payment approach is part of a long-term strategy for better aligning the health care system with a vision of quality. The principal focus of this study is on the Medicare program, as requested, but many of the insights offered in this report are relevant as well to other aspects of the public and private health care sectors.

THE DESIRE TO IMPROVE PERFORMANCE

Americans make large investments in health care every year. In 2004, aggregate spending on health care reached $1.9 trillion, equating to 16 percent of gross domestic product (GDP) and $6,280 per capita (Smith et al., 2006). These figures represent a sevenfold increase over health care expenditures in 1980, and this rapid rate of growth is expected to continue: by 2014, health spending is projected to grow to 18.7 percent of GDP (Heffler et al., 2005).

Several studies of rising health care expenditures have demonstrated that some of these costs are associated with important medical advances, improved health outcomes, and increased value over time (Cutler and Miller, 2005; Murphy and Topel, 2005). For example, both investments in technology and pharmaceutical advances have yielded important gains in longevity. Angioplasty, a treatment for acute myocardial infarction, has been found to yield long-term benefits, such as higher survival rates and better outcomes relative to other, less expensive treatments, such as streptokinase (Zijlstra et al., 1999). Another area in which additional costs are incurred but are associated with important medical advances is prevention of specific cancers through screenings for particular populations, such as Pap smears for cervical cancer, mammography for breast cancer, and use of fecal occult blood testing for colorectal cancer (USPSTF, 2006). Certain treatments, such as hemodialysis, which cost Medicare $14.8 billion in 2003 for approximately 400,000 enrollees (USRDS, 2006), have also been shown to prolong life.

The growth in expenditures and per capita health care spending in the United States far exceeds that in other developed countries. In spite of this spending, the United States still ranks in the bottom quartile of industrialized countries for life expectancy and infant mortality (Hussey et al., 2004). Within the United States, the level of Medicare spending per capita varies twofold from one geographic region to another, and varies even more during the last 6 months of life, without evidence of more effective care or better outcomes in the high-spending areas (Wennberg et al., 2002). Although the health status of Americans generally has improved over time, in some important areas it has not improved significantly or has even deteriorated. For example, obesity has increased dramatically in the population aged 20–74 since the 1980s (NCHS, 2005). During the period 1999–2002, 31 percent of adults were obese, and another 34 percent were overweight. Obesity is a major risk factor for many diseases, including diabetes, which increased in the population aged 20 and older from 8.4 percent in 1988–1994 to 9.4 percent in 1999–2002 (NCHS, 2005). For the population over age 60, the diabetes rate increased from 18.9 to 20.9 percent between the same time frames. The United States lags behind many other countries (where per capita spending levels are lower) in such areas as longevity, heart disease, and diabetes (Schoen et al., 2004; Banks et al., 2006). Statistics such as these have led some analysts to suggest that the current incentive structure creates excessive waste and inefficiency (Skinner et al., 2006) by encouraging complex, expensive, and profitable services that are not necessary to achieve high-quality outcomes, while at the same time discouraging primary care and other services that could yield significant gains (Ginsburg and Grossman, 2005).

The desire to improve performance, encourage patient-centered practices, and deliver high-quality care across provider settings more efficiently has engaged interest in designing payment incentives that might help achieve these goals. Recognizing that much of the increase in health care spending will shift from the private sector and Medicaid to Medicare with the initiation of the Medicare prescription drug benefit (Heffler et al., 2005) and the aging of the baby boomer generation, policy makers and researchers have raised concern about the value received for Medicare dollars. Many policy makers are now seeking to reframe these expenses as public investments that should be designed to leverage higher levels of quality and performance for all Americans (Davis et al., 2005; Davis and Collins, 2006).

CLINICAL QUALITY, PATIENT-CENTEREDNESS, AND EFFICIENCY

Ultimately, pay for performance is one of several mutually reinforcing reform strategies that collectively could move the health care system toward providing better-quality care and improved outcomes. The *Quality Chasm* report identified six fundamental aims associated with health care quality: safety, effectiveness, patient-centeredness, timeliness, efficiency, and equity (IOM, 2001). A broad range of activities is now under way to develop evidence-based measurable standards and outcomes for each of these aims. Many physician specialty societies, trade organizations, and public and private purchasers are developing new performance measures that can provide valuable benchmarks for assessing the quality of care for particular diseases and conditions in various provider settings. As noted above, such performance measures are essential building blocks for any quality improvement effort, including pay for performance.

In addition, patients and their caregivers are becoming more active in managing their care, and are increasingly seeking providers who are sensitive to their needs and preferences, especially in such areas as patient–provider communication, patient experiences with provider services, and attention to care transitions across care settings. New measures have recently emerged that capture these important dimensions of the patient's experience, and such patient-centered measures are becoming more important in consumer evaluations and professional certification of the performance of hospitals, physicians, long-term care facilities, other institutional health care providers, and health plans.

Faced with rapidly growing health insurance premiums and out-of-pocket costs, patients and payers also need measures of efficiency to help them select providers who deliver high-quality care at lower cost. Currently, for example, incentives are often lacking to deter the provision of services of low clinical value and promote the provision of quality services at a lower cost. If health plan purchasers in the public and private sectors are to offer high-quality, affordable health care services, they must have efficiency measures that can be used to develop better payment and performance measurement systems. Despite the importance of measurement, however, effective measures for all six quality aims have not yet been developed.

The committee found it useful to consolidate the six aims into three broad domains when considering what the focus of an initial pay-for-performance strategy should be:

• *Clinical quality*, which encompasses effectiveness, safety, timeliness, and equity.
• *Patient-centeredness*, an attribute of care that reflects the informed preferences of the patient and the patient's significant others, as well as timeliness and equity.
• *Efficiency*, defined as achieving the highest level of quality for a given level of resources.

In assessing pay for performance, the committee explored strategies that could improve performance within each of these three domains, as well as strategies for incorporating these domains into a seamless set of goals for the health care system. The committee recognized the inherent tensions among the three domains. One could strive for high clinical quality and patient-centered care, for example, without being concerned about overall resource use and levels of efficiency. Such an approach could ultimately bankrupt the nation. Conversely, one could emphasize efficiency without accounting adequately for significant variations in clinical quality or patient-centered care. This emphasis could lead to stringent cost containment practices that would compromise the quality of clinical care and patient experiences of care. There is a critical need to achieve an appropriate balance among the three domains that reflects both national values and budgetary constraints.

Recognizing that there is room for provider improvement in all three domains, payment strategies should be aimed at achieving higher performance levels in all three and should also stimulate the development of measures to close existing gaps wherever feasible. Therefore, payment strategies should not be designed to reward high clinical quality alone, but should incorporate incentives to ensure that high-quality care is patient-centered and focused on efficiency as well. Similarly, payment strategies should not be aimed at driving down costs at the expense of patient preferences or clinical quality, but should support an integrated and coordinated system of care that emphasizes improving outcomes through efficient use of resources.

The introduction of payment incentives designed to reward care that is of high clinical quality, patient-centered, and efficient poses daunting challenges. As noted, promising strategies aimed at achieving objectives in one domain may produce adverse or unintended consequences in other domains. Moreover, key components, relationships, and systemwide reforms necessary to achieve the desired goals may be difficult to implement within the vast and diverse array of private and public provider settings that constitute the nation's health care system.

CURRENT STATE OF PAY-FOR-PERFORMANCE EFFORTS

Despite the challenges, many payers, medical groups, and purchasers are currently experimenting with new payment approaches designed to reward higher levels of performance and obtain greater value from health care investments. In the past few years, more than 100 pay-for-performance and incentive programs have been launched in the private sector that offer financial rewards for higher levels of provider performance according to specified measures (Med-Vantage Inc., 2006). Medicare, the nation's largest single payer for health care services, is also experimenting with pay-for-performance strategies through a series of demonstration programs (see Chapter 2) (CMS, 2005b). While many have invested in the promise of pay for performance, however, results are yet to be identified. The impact of these efforts and their effects on provider behavior and patient health may not be realized for many years.

The recent experimentation with pay for performance on the part of private health plans offers an intriguing and attractive potential source of guidance for alternative payment arrangements for traditional Medicare. Experiments such as those implemented within Anthem Blue Cross and Blue Shield and Hawaii's Blue Cross and Blue Shield plan have been operating since 1999. The Integrated Healthcare Association's program covers 8 million enrollees (Epstein et al., 2004). (These and other recent pay-for-performance programs are discussed in Chapter 2.) As pioneering efforts, these programs can offer important models and lessons to inform future health care purchasing or investment strategies in the public sector. (See Chapter 2 for a discussion of early experiences with pay for performance and Appendix B for a summary of the literature on such programs.) To date, however, the results of these early efforts have not been systematically examined, nor have specific factors in success that could help guide the development of pay-for-performance programs been identified. In addition, the evidence base to support pay for performance is still emerging. Fewer than 20 empirical studies have assessed the use of payment incentives to improve quality (Petersen et al., 2006). These studies, focused on improving processes and outcomes of care, access to care, and patient experiences of care in a variety of populations and care settings, have yielded mixed results on the effectiveness of pay-for-performance programs (see Chapter 2).

Thus the ability of pay for performance to achieve the desired goals will be highly dependent on the presence or absence of several key elements not yet determined. Great uncertainty exists about the specific thresholds and preconditions necessary for pay for performance to succeed. Consequently, it is important for pay for performance to be introduced within learning environments that can identify key lessons from early experience and offer the opportunity for midcourse corrections where necessary. Lessons learned and dissemination of best practices could become critical to the development of successful pay-for-performance programs in the absence of a strong evidence base.

As noted above, introducing pay-for-performance strategies within Medicare poses numerous challenges. Unavoidable decisions will have to be made that will reward some providers and penalize others. To achieve higher levels of performance throughout the health care system, strong public- and private-sector partnerships and new governmental arrangements will be necessary. New measures of performance will have to be developed. More important, ongoing monitoring and evaluation will be essential. Independent and objective research focused on early experiences will be required to (1) identify key areas in which new payment strategies can make important differences, (2) explore the necessary resource and implementation costs, and (3) resolve multiple uncertainties and stakeholder disputes that will emerge along the way.

OVERVIEW OF THE MEDICARE PROGRAM

To understand the nuances of implementing pay for performance in Medicare, it is necessary to understand the basics of the program. Medicare is the government health program for the U.S. elderly population (those over age 65) and those who are eligible because of permanent kidney failure or suffer from a long-term disability. The program, which covered nearly 42 million Americans in 2004—35.4 million elderly and 6.3 million disabled (CMS, 2005a)—is financed through beneficiary premiums and federal general revenues and payroll taxes. Although Medicare is administered by the Centers for Medicare and Medicaid Services (CMS), a federal agency, beneficiaries are served almost entirely through the private-sector health care delivery system (MedPAC, 2005b).

Medicare consists of four components:

• Part A, the Hospital Insurance program, pays on a fee-for-service basis for inpatient hospital care and some home health, skilled nursing facility, and hospice services.

- Part B covers, also on a fee-for-service basis, outpatient hospital, home health, physician, and other individual health care provider services, as well as such services as clinical laboratory and diagnostic tests, supplies, and durable medical equipment.
- Part C, or Medicare Advantage (formerly Medicare+Choice), provides capitated payments to private plans that agree to provide Medicare beneficiaries with the services covered by Parts A and B. It offers beneficiaries an expanded choice of delivery systems, including various forms of managed care, such as health maintenance organizations and preferred provider organizations.
- Part D, first implemented in 2006, provides coverage for therapeutic drugs through private health insurance plans.

Medicare expenditures in 2004 amounted to more than $300 billion, 16.5 percent of the total national health expenditures of $1,878 billion (see Table 1-1). In that year, federal health expenditures, excluding federal employees' health benefits, came to $600 billion, 32.6 percent of total national health expenditures (CMS, 2006). Over the last three decades, Medicare spending has grown at a faster rate than the balance of all national health expenditures (see Table 1-1), although on a per beneficiary basis, expenditures have grown somewhat more slowly than those covered under private insurance (Davis and Collins, 2006).

Medicare contracts with private providers for the provision of services to its beneficiaries, for which it pays according to agreed-upon payment rates and methodologies. Unlike private insurers, which often contract

TABLE 1-1 Estimated Medicare and National Health Expenditures, 1975–2004

Expenditures	1975 (billions of dollars)	1985 (billions of dollars)	1995 (billions of dollars)	2004 (billions of dollars)	Increase 1975–2004 (percent)
Medicare	16.3	71.4	182.4	309.0	1,796
National health expenditures	133.6	441.9	1,020.4	1,877.6	1,305
Medicare expenditures as percentage of national health expenditures	12.2	16.2	17.9	16.5	35

SOURCE: CMS, 2006.

selectively with available providers, Medicare has traditionally allowed all licensed providers to participate in the program who (1) wish to serve Medicare beneficiaries, (2) are willing to accept Medicare's administratively set rates as payment, and (3) meet minimal predetermined federal standards. Each provider setting has its own requirements for Medicare participation. Essentially all institutional providers must undergo accreditation or certification by CMS or its agents, and many report performance data. For example, hospitals are required to develop and maintain a quality assessment and performance improvement program, meet standards for content and retention of medical records, and fulfill requirements for organization and functioning of medical staff, among many other conditions. Participating physicians must agree to accept Medicare's payment for covered services as the full charge and not bill the Medicare patient for additional fees above the applicable coinsurance or deductible. While most doctors "accept assignment" as participating physicians, others do not and can bill a limited amount above the Medicare payment. All physicians billing Medicare, nonetheless, agree to specific billing procedures. There are, however, no quality or performance requirements for physicians to participate in Medicare beyond state licensure.

Medicare payments have historically been made on the basis of standard formulas or fee schedules that do not reflect different levels of performance (see Appendix A). This payment system was based on the assumption that all licensed providers who met the conditions of participation would provide care of acceptable quality. This payment approach generally persists today, even though it is now recognized that significant variations exist in the quality of care offered by providers and that the average level of care is far from that associated with current best practices. (See Chapter 2 for more discussion of payment systems.)

Current Medicare care payment practices can have toxic effects because they do not reflect the relative value of certain services, such as preventive and primary care, and place little or no emphasis on achieving high levels of clinical quality within a given amount of resources. For example, the physician's fee schedule does not pay providers adequately for cognitive services such as care coordination and patient education, which are essential for patients with chronic conditions. In addition, the data and methodologies that CMS uses to calculate certain payments under the physician's fee schedule tend to favor relatively new high-technology services (MedPAC, 2006). Costs are frequently driven upward by a system that provides incentives for a high volume of services, but not for efforts to promote the basic principles of higher-quality care. The system also encourages utilization of expensive services that may not be more effective than less costly ones. In fact, the fee-for-service system itself, as well as the payment methodology for various providers, encourages an increase in quantity and intensity of services. Medicare's hospital outpatient payment system and that for physicians and other health care professionals tend to pay for each additional service, even if the service results from a complication or inadequate initial service. Thus, a provider who makes a mistake and has to repeat a procedure may be paid twice as much as one who performs it correctly the first time. Payment systems that bundle services broadly and comprehensively into a single payment run the risk of having providers avoid patients with extensive needs that are not adequately accounted for in the payment. For example, patients requiring extensive care in a skilled nursing facility can have relatively long waits for placement in such a facility because the base payment does not reflect all their likely needs (MedPAC, 2005a). Medicare's various prospective payment systems and their incentives are discussed in Appendix A.

Just as payment methodologies can have an impact on the quality of health care, there are other aspects of the current health care delivery system that may affect care. For example, consumer-directed health plans are based on the expectation that greater transparency about service costs and quality and a greater responsibility for paying for care, including tiered benefit levels, will motivate consumers to select their health care providers carefully, which in turn will motivate providers to improve their efficiency and clinical performance in order to attract patients. Such health plans are relatively new and their full impact has yet to be measured, but they may have a positive influence on health costs and quality in the future.

Another way to overcome the unintended consequences of the current payment system is to create incentives to promote better quality through pay-for-performance strategies. Such strategies reward outcomes and processes associated with improved and/or high-quality care according to selected measures of provider performance. The committee recognizes that such a reward strategy will not necessarily result in lower spending for health care services, but improving quality should make it more likely that patients will receive more effective and efficient care. Although the promise of pay for performance may alter provider behaviors, it alone will not be the silver bullet for achieving high-quality care or curbing health care costs; it will, however, help ensure that what is paid for will be more helpful to patients.

The long-term growth in Medicare expenditures is projected to be substantial (see Table 1-2), creating a significant impetus for the development of payment strategies that can provide incentives for efficiency while encouraging high levels of clinical quality and patient-centered care. Because Medicare is such a large payer and because many private payers follow its policy lead, the program exerts a significant influence on the organization and delivery of health care services throughout the United States. Through its coverage and payment decisions, therefore, it could encourage the diffusion of high-quality practices.

TABLE 1-2   Estimated and Projected Medicare Spending (billions of dollars)

	1975	1985	1995	2005[a]	2014[a]
Part A	10.6	48.7	114.9	179.9[b]	317.8
Part B	4.2	22.7	65.2	151.3	261.2
Part D	—	—	—	1.7	169.0
Total	14.8	71.4	180.1	332.9	748.0

[a]Intermediate estimates.
[b]Shifts in funding for some home health care from Part A to Part B are reflected in the relative spending in 2005.
SOURCE: Boards of Trustees, Federal Hospital Insurance and Federal Supplementary Medical Insurance Trust Funds, 2005.

INITIAL STEPS TO IMPROVE THE U.S. HEALTH CARE SYSTEM

As noted earlier, the introduction of pay for performance needs to be examined within a framework of evolving measures and shifting organizational structures and collaborations throughout the health care system. The ability to implement pay for performance is not distributed evenly across all health care settings. Some organizations, such as hospitals and certain specialty practices, have acquired extensive experience with performance measures and quality improvement. Others, most notably individual providers and many primary care settings, are just beginning to experiment systematically with quality improvement measures and strategies.

Recognizing that reforms are necessary, leaders in health care and government are considering alternative approaches to implementing a pay-for-performance strategy. One option is to allow quality improvement processes to evolve at a gradual pace, driven by motivated purchasers and providers, and implemented through scattered local experiments with new payment strategies in selected systems of care or geographic regions. This approach can reveal the opportunities and challenges involved in introducing new measures and performance-based care in the treatment of selected health conditions in different care settings. While this approach may generate important insights about the promise and limitations of payment strategies, however, it may be insufficient to achieve the breadth and scope of change necessary to influence provider behavior and practices. It also may fail to identify the key payment incentives and other environmental features necessary to change practices among low performers or poor-quality health care settings if they do not volunteer to participate.

A second option is to restructure the Medicare payment system to encourage more rapid transformation and to foster national systemwide change. Such an approach could apply the level of resources necessary to achieve significant changes in practices and collaborative arrangements, which may vary with the severity and complexity of clinical conditions and the performance measures employed. Yet restructuring the payment system in the absence of reliable evidence of positive outcomes associated with new payment incentives poses substantial risks. Certain unknown system requirements may be necessary to ensure that pay-for-performance strategies have their intended effects and do not have unintended adverse consequences. Key features and adjustments must be considered, such as how performance measures will address patients with multiple chronic diseases when accepted measures of high-quality care for one condition may contradict measures of high-quality care for another. If payment strategies are not carefully aligned with desired outcomes, providers may avoid accepting patients whose conditions would jeopardize their performance or withdraw from the Medicare system entirely. Both providers in organizational settings (such as hospitals and skilled nursing facilities) and solo practitioners will need data tools and quality improvement assistance to comply with reporting requirements that will allow them to participate in a pay-for-performance program.

In this report, the committee seeks to weigh these two approaches through an evidence-based analysis, keeping in mind that the current payment systems continue to have negative unintended consequences (discussed in Appendix A). The committee proposes a multiphase approach within a learning environment aimed at achieving transformation through a series of structured changes in current payment arrangements. The committee also examines the core features necessary to implement a pay-for-performance strategy while respecting the need for variation and tailored approaches in different health care environments.

CONCLUSIONS

Changes in the structure of Medicare payments could have a major impact on the quality of care delivered by the entire health care delivery system. As Medicare provides health care benefits to nearly 42 million U.S. citizens at an annual cost of well over $300 billion (2004 expenditures), CMS is in a unique position to lead the American health care industry in providing higher-quality care and greater value for the money spent on that care (IOM, 2002). Medicare's current payment system is often inconsistent with the goal of promoting higher value. Some in the private sector have moved forward with attempts to reform the current payment system, but these efforts will not realize their maximum benefit without public-sector involvement. Medicare is also working on strategies to add value to the care it provides and is now collaborating with the private sector to accelerate change.

Notwithstanding the difficulties involved in overhauling the current payment system and the gaps and uncertainties in the existing evidence base for pay for performance, the committee believes pay for performance could be a viable tool when used in tandem with other performance improvement strategies, such as public reporting and technical assistance, to transform the health care delivery system. The ultimate purpose of a performance-based payment system is to stimulate behavioral and organizational change within the provider community in ways that will foster performance improvement and improve the value of health care services. The committee does not presume that these changes will be easy or that savings will automatically be generated. It also remains cognizant of the unintended consequences that could arise, but believes the consequences of inaction pose a greater threat.

The lack of evidence associating pay for performance with improvements in clinical quality, patient-centeredness, efficiency, and, most important, outcomes of care suggests that caution will be necessary as Medicare proceeds. The consequences of aligning incentives to promote higher-quality health care are largely unknown. For instance, providers might avoid treating high-risk, nonadherent, or other types of patients who could jeopardize their performance scores. Payment rewards might encourage a system in which providers would work to improve only on measures for which they were paid, and as a consequence, reduce their quality of care on unrewarded measures instead of trying to improve care on a more global level. From the patient's perspective, payment incentives could undermine the revered physician–patient relationships, which are based largely on trust. A pay-for-performance program could also increase competition within the health care enterprise and thereby impede knowledge transfer among providers. Recognizing the need for some kind of payment reform and the promise of pay for performance as suggested by early experiments in the private sector, it will be necessary to balance actions taken toward implementation of the approach with due caution. This report therefore emphasizes the need to introduce pay for performance within a comprehensive learning system through a multiphase approach that addresses significant variations in clinical conditions and health care settings, and encompasses an evaluation strategy for deriving insights from the experience gained in early stages of implementation.

SCOPE AND ORGANIZATION OF THE REPORT

This report sets forth a vision for how pay for performance could be implemented to best help achieve the goals of improving health care quality and patient outcomes. While the report outlines options, designers should not be limited to these options; rather, the report is intended to delineate principles for the development of performance-based rewards.

Chapter 2 reviews the promise of pay for performance as assessed in research studies and suggested by initial experiments, while also exploring its potential unintended adverse consequences. Chapter 3 reviews options for funding a pay-for-performance program for Medicare. Chapters 4 and 5, respectively, provide an overview of various reward distribution options and present the committee's proposed multiphase approach to the implementation of a comprehensive pay-for-performance program. Finally, an aggressive research and evaluation agenda and key features of the kind of learning system the committee believes should be the context for the introduction of pay for performance are detailed in Chapter 6.

REFERENCES

Banks J, Marmot M, Oldfield Z, Smith JP. 2006. Disease and disadvantage in the United States and in England. *Journal of the American Medical Association* 295(17):2037–2045.

Boards of Trustees of the Federal Hospital Insurance and Federal Supplementary Medical Insurance Trust Funds. 2005. *2005 Annual Report of the Boards of Trustees of the Federal Hospital Insurance and Federal Supplementary Medical Insurance Trust Funds.* Washington, DC: Medicare Board of Trustees.

CMS (Centers for Medicare and Medicaid Services). 2005a. *Medicare Information Resource.* [Online]. Available: http://www.cms.hhs.gov/medicare/ [accessed December 6, 2005].

CMS. 2005b. *Medicare "Pay for Performance (P4P)" Initiatives.* [Online]. Available: http://www.cms.hhs.gov/apps /media/press/release.asp?counter=1343 [accessed June 13, 2006].

CMS. 2006. *National Health Expenditures by Type of Service and Source of Funds.* [Online]. Available: http://www.cms.hhs.gov/NationalHealthExpendData/02_NationalHealth Accounts Historical.asp#TopofPage [accessed April, 18, 2006].

Cutler D, Miller G. 2005. The role of public health improvements in health advances: The twentieth-century United States. *Demography* 42(1):1–22.

Davis K, Collins S. 2006. Medicare at forty. *Health Care Financing Review 2005–2006* 27(2):53–62.

Davis K, Schoenbaum S, Audet A. 2005. A 2020 vision of patient-centered primary care. *Journal of General Internal Medicine* 20(10):953–967.

Epstein AM, Lee TH, Hamel MB. 2004. Paying physicians for high-quality care. *New England Journal of Medicine* 350(4):406–410.

Fisher ES, Wennberg DE, Stukel TA, Gottlieb DJ. 2004. Variations in the longitudinal efficiency of academic medical centers. *Health Affairs* VAR19–VAR32.

Ginsburg PB, Grossman JM. 2005. When the price isn't right: How inadvertent payment incentives drive medical care. *Health Affairs* w5.376.

Heffler S, Smith S, Keehan S, Borger C, Clemens MK, Truffer C. 2005. Trends: U.S. health spending projections for 2004–2014. *Health Affairs* w5.74.

Hussey PS, Anderson GF, Osborn R, Feek C, McLaughlin V, Millar J, Epstein A. 2004. How does the quality of care compare in five countries? *Health Affairs* 3(23):89–99.

IOM (Institute of Medicine). 2000. *To Err Is Human: Building a Safer Health System.* Kohn LT, Corrigan JM, Donaldson MS, eds. Washington, DC: National Academy Press.

IOM. 2001. *Crossing the Quality Chasm: A New Health System for the 21st Century.* Washington, DC: National Academy Press.

IOM. 2002. *Leadership by Example: Coordinating Government Roles in Improving Health Care Quality*. Corrigan JM, Eden J, Smith BM, eds. Washington, DC: The National Academies Press.

IOM. 2006a. *Medicare's Quality Improvement Organization Program: Maximizing Potential*. Washington, DC: The National Academies Press.

IOM. 2006b. *Performance Measurement: Accelerating Improvement*. Washington, DC: The National Academies Press.

Leape LL, Berwick DM. 2005. Five years after To Err Is Human: What have we learned? *Journal of the American Medical Association* 293(19):2384–2390.

Med-Vantage Inc. 2006. *Pay for Performance*. [Online]. Available: http://medvantageinc.com/Content/solutions.p4p.php4 [accessed June 9, 2006].

MedPAC (Medicare Payment Advisory Commission). 2005a. *Report to the Congress: Medicare Payment Policy*. Washington, DC: MedPAC.

MedPAC. 2005b. *Report to the Congress: Medicare Payment Policy*. [Online]. Available: http://www.medpac.gov/publications/congressional_reports/Mar05_TOC.pdf [accessed December 6, 2005].

MedPAC. 2006. *Report to Congress: Increasing the Value of Medicare*. Washington, DC: MedPAC.

Murphy K, Topel R. 2005. *The Value of Health and Longevity*. Cambridge, MA: National Bureau of Economic Research.

NCHS (National Center for Health Statistics). 2005. *Health, United States, 2005: With Chartbook Trends in the Health of Americans*. Hyattsville, MD: U.S. Government Printing Office.

Petersen LA, Woodard LD, Urech T, Daw C, Sookanan S. 2006. Does pay-for-performance improve the quality of health care? *Annals of Internal Medicine* 145(4):265–272.

Schoen C, Osborn R, Huynh PT, Doty M, Davis K, Zapert K, Peugh J. 2004. Primary care and health system performance: Adults' experiences in five countries. *Health Affairs* w4.487.

Skinner JS, Staiger DO, Fisher ES. 2006. Is technological change in medicine always worth it? The case of acute myocardial infarction. *Health Affairs* 25.w34.

Smith C, Cowan C, Heffler S, Catlin A, National Health Accounts Team. 2006. National health spending in 2004: Recent slowdown led by prescription drug spending. *Health Affairs* 25(1):186–196.

USPSTF (U.S. Preventive Services Task Force). 2006. *Guide to Clinical Preventive Services*. [Online]. Available: http://www.ahrq.gov/clinic/cps.3dix.htm [accessed June 13, 2006].

USRDS (United States Renal Data System). 2006. *2005 Annual Data Report: Atlas of End Stage Renal Disease in the United States*. [Online]. Available: http://www.usrds.org/adr.htm [accessed May 27, 2006].

Wennberg JE, Fisher ES, Skinner JS. 2002. Geography and the debate over Medicare reform. *Health Affairs* w2.96.

Zijlstra F, Hoorntje JCA, de Boer M-J, Reiffers S, Miedema K, Ottervanger JP, van't Hof AW, Suryapranata H. 1999. Long-term benefit of primary angioplasty as compared with thrombolytic therapy for acute myocardial infarction. *New England Journal of Medicine* 341(19):1413–1419.

2

The Promise of Pay for Performance

CHAPTER SUMMARY

This chapter reviews the current health care payment systems; the strengths, weaknesses, and potential adverse consequences of pay for performance; early experiences with the approach; and the ways in which pay for performance can be used as a pathway to reform. Multiple and complex challenges confront any such effort, and monitoring and evaluation will be essential so stakeholders can learn from experience, identify unanticipated consequences, and implement midcourse adjustments as necessary.

Current payment systems are not well aligned with efforts to achieve the six quality aims set forth in the Quality Chasm *report (IOM, 2001). These systems place little emphasis on achieving high clinical quality, do not reflect the value of services, frequently act to drive up costs, and do not encourage patient-centered care or the efficient use of resources. While this report does not attempt to address all shortcomings of the current systems, the committee's analysis should be viewed within the broader framework of the need for fundamental reform of the health care payment structure.*

The initiatives proposed in this report would modify current health care payment systems by using financial incentives to promote higher levels of quality across diverse health care settings. These initiatives are predicated on the assumption that the health care Americans receive could and should be of considerably greater value—better-quality care obtained at a sustainable and socially acceptable cost (see Chapter 1). Based on a review of the available evidence, the committee concluded that modest changes alone in the current systems—systems in which provider reimbursement is based largely on the quantity of health care services rendered—are unlikely to promote significant progress toward the goals of improved quality and reduced growth in costs. Rather, a profound and fundamental alignment of incentives (financial, informational, and reputational) with desired outcomes is required to stimulate the needed transformational change in the current health care payment systems.

CURRENT PAYMENT SYSTEMS

At present, the care for 88 percent of Medicare beneficiaries, or approximately 35 million individuals, is paid for under fee-for-service systems. The remaining 12 percent of beneficiaries are enrolled in the Medicare Advantage program, under which private plans are paid monthly, risk-adjusted capitated amounts in return for providing Medicare's benefits to those who choose to enroll in Medicare Advantage (Kaiser Family Foundation, 2005). Medicare's fee-for-service payment rates and fees are set administratively by the Centers for Medicare and Medicaid Services (CMS) at levels intended to cover the cost of the resources typically required to provide a particular service. The service may be defined narrowly, such as a chest x-ray, or broadly to encompass a bundle of services, such as all the inpatient hospital care associated with a stay of any duration for a heart bypass operation.

Medicare's rates and fees do not vary with the quality of the service provided. Furthermore, the fee-for-service payment structure generally does not provide reimbursement for health services that are recognized as important contributors to quality, such as comprehensive case management, care coordination, health counseling, and many preventive services that may reduce the need for hospitalization or more expensive future medical procedures. In addition, because of the way payment rates for different services are set relative to one another, new, complex, high-tech interventions tend to be better compensated than procedures involving less intensive service use, less or older technology, and more time with patients (which may be important to quality care) (Ginsburg and Grossman, 2005). Additionally, payment rates and fees do not vary according to the need for a particular service. For example, one study that examined clinical decision making under different payment systems found that expenditures for discretionary services were lower under capitated than under traditional fee-for-service arrangements (Shen et al., 2004). Providers are paid more for doing more and are not penalized when the provided services are of little or no value or, worse yet, negatively affect health outcomes. In some cases, the incentives embodied in fee-for-service payments may encourage the delivery of unnecessary or even harmful services that can raise fundamental concerns about cost and safety (Robinson, 2001).

Since fee-for-service payments offer little direct incentive to improve quality or avoid low-value services, they fall short of fostering goals in the three critical domains identified in Chapter 1: clinical quality, patient-centeredness, and efficiency. Although fee for service is responsive to patient demand for services in the sense that the health care system is responsive to the sickest patients who require more complex and higher levels of care, this type of payment structure offers no incentives to providers or patients to improve overall health status through preventive services or lower-cost interventions that can ultimately reduce the demand for more complex clinical services. The systems pay for treating illness and injury, not for keeping people well.

Since Medicare's inception, policy makers have been concerned about the rapid growth of health care expenditures. The program's payment systems have been modified in response to these concerns, but these changes have not been sufficient. More recently, concern has also focused on the quality of care, and some steps to improve quality have been taken. CMS is currently conducting demonstrations to test payment systems designed to reward higher-quality care, but these initiatives have not yet been implemented on a wide scale. A brief review of Medicare payment policies follows.

Original Medicare Retrospective Payment Systems

Initially, Medicare payment policies followed the prevailing private-sector practice of the early 1960s, which was to reimburse providers for the lesser of either their usual and customary charges or their actual costs for each service delivered. The reimbursement system was retrospective because payments could not be calculated until after the service had been provided; the physician or hospital would not learn the exact payment amount until after the end of the year, when customary charges and actual costs could be audited and payment rates calculated. This payment system provided no real restraint on expenditures. The more providers spent on a service or increased charges, the more Medicare would ultimately pay. To limit growth in expenditures, Medicare began to define more narrowly which costs were acceptable and which were not, as well as to set limits on allowable increases, thereby making the payment system increasingly complex.

Prospective Payment Systems

In an attempt to gain better control over burgeoning expenditures, policy makers began in the 1980s to shift Medicare from retrospective to prospective payment systems. Prospective payment was first introduced in inpatient acute care hospitals in 1983. Since then, CMS has instituted prospective payment for other provider settings, including skilled nursing facilities in 1998, home health agencies in 2000, and outpatient acute care hospitals in 2000 (SUNY, 2001; CMS, 2006c). Physicians are reimbursed according to the Medicare Physician Fee Schedule. The new systems set payments for various services (or bundles of services) in advance of their delivery. Thus, providers know how much they will be paid before they treat their patients and can better plan their care and resource use.

Fees and payment rates of Medicare's prospective payment systems are set administratively to cover CMS's estimate of the average cost of providing a service, plus a small margin. In some instances, the payment does not cover the provider's costs; in other cases, the payment is more than sufficient. In some situations in which costs far exceed payments, Medicare provides additional "outlier payments" that cover a portion of the excess costs. Under most of Medicare's prospective payment systems, payments are adjusted for geographic differences in labor and other costs. In general, prospective payment encourages providers to keep the costs of services below the payment amount and creates incentives to treat those with the least severe and complex conditions in any particular diagnosis, service, or risk category.

As noted above, the unit for which payments are made may be a bundle that encompasses all of the inputs necessary to provide a stay in an institution or perform a procedure, or it may be a discrete, narrowly defined item, test, or service. Under most of the payment systems, unless Congress intervenes, rates are automatically adjusted upward each year based on indexes of anticipated price increases. A major exception is the Medicare Physician Fee Schedule update, which is governed by the sustainable growth rate (SGR). This formula limits the growth in per beneficiary Medicare Physician Fee Schedule expenditures to the growth in per capita gross domestic product. Because the volume and average intensity of services paid for under the Medicare Physician Fee Schedule have been growing very rapidly, application of the SGR formula has resulted in negative updates for physicians in recent years. With the exception of 2002, Congress has acted to avert these reductions (U.S. GAO, 2005). CMS projects that the SGR will impose annual negative updates of more than 4 percent each year during 2007–2011, which may affect physicians' willingness to consider performance-related payment changes and incentives (MedPAC, 2006).

Appendix A presents more detailed descriptions of payment systems and their incentives for in- and outpatient hospital care, skilled nursing facilities, home health care, outpatient dialysis services, physicians, and Medicare Advantage plans. The discussion there is intended to give a broad overview of payment methodologies, not a detailed picture of all the complexities of each method, to provide a context for the consideration of payment incentives. Table 2-1 presents an overall picture of spending in the Medicare program by provider setting.

TABLE 2-1   Medicare Program Spending by Provider Setting, 2003

Setting	Hospital Insurance (billions of dollars)	Supplementary Medical Insurance (billions of dollars)	Total (billions of dollars)	Percent of Total
Hospital	109.4	17.9	127.3	45
Physicians	N/A	48.3	48.3	17
Managed care	19.5	17.2	36.8	13
Skilled nursing facility	14.3	N/A	14.3	5
Home health	2.6	7.1	9.7	3
Other	6.3	33.3	39.6	14

NOTE: N/A = not applicable.
SOURCE: Based on data from MedPAC (MedPAC, 2005).

PAY FOR PERFORMANCE AS A PATHWAY TO REFORM

Pay for performance has emerged as a promising strategy to address the inadequacies of the current payment system outlined above, and has attracted considerable attention in the private marketplace. Additionally, CMS has begun to invest resources in pay for performance as a reform strategy (CMS, 2006a). These pay-for-performance initiatives must be implemented successfully, both to achieve their particular goals—improved quality of care and cost containment—and to prompt the fundamental changes needed in the health care system overall.

In other sectors of the American economy, a reform of this magnitude would be based not only on sound theory, but also on pertinent practical experience. While the database on which to base the design and evaluation of pay-for-performance programs is growing steadily, it remains incomplete and without substantial validation. Despite this lack of a definitive evidence base, both private- and public-sector decision makers would like to move forward aggressively with pay-for-performance programs. However, experience with other health care initiatives suggests that the rapid implementation of new payment strategies based on theory and preliminary results does not always achieve the desired goals. In fact, it can prove to be counterproductive, exacerbating current problems and creating new ones.

The Theory Behind Pay for Performance

In essence, pay for performance represents an attempt to align incentives in the payment system so that rewards are given to providers who foster the six quality aims set forth in the *Quality Chasm* report (IOM,

2001) (see Chapter 1) and improve health outcomes while using resources parsimoniously. At the most basic level, improving care requires changes in the behavior of providers. Paying providers for improving performance or achieving superior levels of performance should motivate them to focus on doing so in measured areas. Pay for performance also has the potential to achieve change by influencing the environment in which providers practice. For instance, performance-based payment could make it attractive for both providers and provider organizations to invest in improved systems for tracking and enhancing the quality of care, making them better able to manage the health of the populations they serve. Ideally, pay for performance would encourage certain changes in structural and organizational practices, such as a new emphasis on comprehensive and coordinated care and collaboration across individual settings of care, and stimulate consumers to pay attention to quality practices.

Effects of Medicare Payment Systems on Provider Behavior

Evidence that providers have responded to changes in Medicare payment policies in the past suggests that health care providers will likely change their behavior in response to Medicare payment incentives to improve quality. The implementation of various Medicare prospective payment systems has been associated with significant changes in provider behavior. All of these behavior changes cannot be attributed conclusively to the new payment systems because those systems did not emerge in isolation, and because research on their effects often examined varying aspects of change, used different data, and focused on different types of providers. Nonetheless, the literature attests to dramatic shifts in the way health care is delivered since the new systems were instituted. For example:

- In the 1980s, hospital discharges and average lengths of stay were slowly decreasing among those under age 65, while both rates were increasing for the Medicare population. This trend reversed in the Medicare population after a prospective payment system was implemented in acute care hospitals in 1983. Also, utilization rates dropped dramatically in 1984 and 1985, while those rates among the rest of the population continued to decrease at a more gradual pace, although utilization increased somewhat for both populations later in the 1980s (Hodgkin and McGuire, 1994).
- Controlled studies of the responses of hospitals to Medicare payment changes showed that their behavior was related directly to Medicare's portion of their volume. Thus hospitals that were more dependent on Medicare patients were likely to show a larger change in the observed behavior relative to hospitals with a smaller proportion of Medicare patients (Hodgkin and McGuire, 1994).

• One study that compared cost-based and flat-rate Medicaid payments for skilled nursing facilities and intermediate care facilities found that facilities in states with cost-based reimbursement tended to have more registered nurses and fewer licensed practical nurses per resident than facilities in flat-rate states, regardless of the ownership status of the facility (Cohen and Spector, 1996).

• A nursing home study based on Medicare claims data and other administrative datasets examined the charges of skilled nursing facilities for rehabilitation therapy (physical, occupational, and speech therapies) (White, 2003). When a prospective payment system was implemented, there was a dramatic drop in the percentage of skilled nursing facility residents that received a high level of therapy (more than $200/day), and residents of these facilities were more likely to receive a moderate level of daily therapy than either extremely high levels or no therapy. The changes observed were consistent with the incentives of the prospective payment system, which offers relatively generous payments for moderate levels of rehabilitation therapy and stops paying for therapy above a specified level per week. The changes were observed between 1997 and 2000. Transition to the new payment system was gradual, beginning in 1998.

Early Experiences with Pay for Performance

Public-Sector Efforts

CMS has undertaken several Medicare pay-for-performance initiatives for different provider settings. Some of these initiatives are in the planning phase; others have recently been implemented. One example of the latter is CMS's demonstration project with Premier, Inc. (the Premier Hospital Quality Incentive Demonstration), in which hospitals among the top 20 percent of performers receive bonus payments (CMS, 2006b; Premier Inc., 2006). Year 1 of the project yielded positive results among the 262 participating hospitals; data showed statistically significant improvement in all five clinical areas examined, with an overall improvement of 6.6 percent (Remus, 2005). Another such project is Medicare's Physician Group Practice Demonstration, which rewards group practices for their performance on quality-of-care metrics, but only after the practices achieve savings of at least 2 percent of projected expenditures (Kautter et al., 2004).

Other CMS projects in development focus on promoting the adoption and use of information technologies among physicians and the use of disease management models to improve the quality of care. Bonuses (or administrative fees) are often contingent upon demonstration of net savings to Medicare. The 3-year Medicare Management Performance Demonstration was mandated by the Medicare Prescription Drug, Improvement, and Modernization Act of 2003. The project focuses on small and medium-sized physician practices, and promotes the use of health information technologies to improve care for the chronically ill. The same act also mandated several disease management projects that often make vendor fees dependent on proven savings.

CMS is currently running several other demonstrations that include projects related to dialysis facilities, nursing homes, and chronic care (CMS, 2006a). While the demonstrations are impressive in number and variety and may yield valuable insights, demonstration projects in and of themselves may not generate large changes in the health care system since they tend to be short-lived, end with isolated reports to Congress, and do not necessarily lead to specific follow-up activities.

Aside from these specific efforts, it is important to note that CMS is actively collaborating with the Ambulatory care Quality Alliance and the Hospital Quality Alliance on pay-for-performance strategies. This type of collaboration is key to the success of pay for performance, not only for the improvement of individual programs through shared learning, but also for the success of pay for performance on a larger level through alignment of incentives, decreased confusion associated with multiple requirements, and synergism among the multiple efforts under way.

Private-Sector Efforts

In the past several years, numerous employers, purchasing coalitions, and health plans have announced new efforts to reward health care quality. Estimates suggest that more than 100 individual pay-for-performance efforts are currently under way (Med-Vantage Inc., 2006). These programs vary in the number and types (e.g., process or outcome) of quality indicators used, the clinical conditions targeted, the magnitude of the incentives and how they are structured (e.g., as a competition in which only the top providers receive a bonus or as an award based on performance relative to a common benchmark), and whether the program applies to a large or small share of a provider's patients. Several examples are described below to illustrate the diversity of approaches.

In California, seven health plans are coordinating pay-for-performance programs under the auspices of the Integrated Healthcare Association (IHA), a multistakeholder coalition (www.iha.org). The seven plans consist of 225 physician groups representing about 35,000 physicians treating 6.2 million patients (IHA, 2006a). Bonuses are awarded to large, multispecialty physician groups based on clinical process measures from the Health Plan Employer Data and Information Set (HEDIS), patient experiences of care,

TABLE 2-2   IHA Pay for Performance 2006 Measurement Set

Domain	Measure (measurement year 2006, reporting year 2007)	Weight
Clinical	1. Childhood immunizations	50%
	2. Childhood upper respiratory infection (appropriate treatment)	
	3. Cervical cancer screening	
	4. Breast cancer screening	
	5. Asthma (use of appropriate medication)	
	6. Diabetes: HbA_1c screening	
	7. Diabetes: HbA_1c control	
	8. Cholesterol: LDL screening	
	9. Cholesterol: LDL control <130	
	10. Chlamydia screening	
	11. Nephropathy monitoring for diabetic patients	
Patient Experience	1. Specialty care	30%
	2. Timely access to care	
	3. Doctor–patient communication	
	4. Overall ratings of care	
	5. Care coordination	
Information Technology Investment	1. Integrate clinical electronic datasets at group level	20%
	2. Support clinical decision making at point of care	
	(Each activity is worth 5%. The maximum 20% credit requires four activities, at least two of which must be from measure 2.)	

SOURCE: IHA, 2006a.

and investments in technology and infrastructure. Table 2-2 lists the specific measures targeted for IHA's 2006 program (the fourth year of the program) in three domains and the weights used to determine the share of the total possible bonus that is allocated to each domain. While performance measures are common across the seven plans, the structure of the bonus varies; most plans have opted to reward only the top performers (e.g., the top deciles or quartiles) using a bonus that is proportional to the number of the plan's patients cared for by the group. Additionally, for the 2006 measurement/2007 reporting year, IHA encourages health plans to reward year-to-year improvement (IHA, 2006b).

Some large employers, through coalitions, are also beginning to offer direct rewards for physician performance on health care quality measures. One example is Bridges to Excellence (www.bridgestoexcellence.org), which operates in four markets and involves a collaborative effort among several large employers, including General Electric and Verizon Communications. Bridges to Excellence offers physicians who become certified by the Diabetes Physician Recognition Program[1] $100 for each diabetic patient in their panel. This program requires physicians to document performance on a number of process and outcome measures through medical record review. Similarly, the Heart/Stroke Physician Recognition Program[2] has been launched in selected markets. Finally, through Physician Practice Connections,[3] doctors can receive up to $55 per patient for establishing clinical information systems in their offices that aid in regular follow-up for chronically ill patients and for implementing patient education programs.

Pay-for-performance programs are being used in both the health maintenance organization (HMO) and preferred provider organization (PPO) settings. Since 1999, the Hawaii Medical Service Association, the local Blue Cross and Blue Shield affiliated plan and the largest health plan in the state, has rewarded the physicians in its PPO network based on quality measures. In 2003, individual bonuses ranged from $500 to $20,000 (Landro, 2004). These bonuses represent about 5.5 percent of the physician's overall salary (Rosenthal et al., 2004). Anthem Blue Cross and Blue Shield of New Hampshire's plan pays bonuses based on a variety of measures that assess appropriate primary and secondary prevention, including screening for breast, cervical, and prostate cancer; screening of patients with coronary artery disease for high cholesterol; and provision of retinal exams for diabetic patients. Anthem's performance bonus was $20 per patient per year for the top quartile of physicians (about 5 percent of compensation) and about half of that amount for physicians ranked between the 50th and 75th percentiles. Physicians were also eligible for an additional payment of $20 per patient for participating in the plan's disease management program (Rosenthal et al., 2004).

Some medical groups and independent practice associations incorporate incentive programs into their payment methods. For example, the Hill Physicians Medical Group, one of the nation's largest independent practice associations, puts up to 15 percent of physician compensation at risk based on quality performance (PBGH, 2005). The program looks at clinical measures (including IHA measures plus other HEDIS measures), information technology functionality, and patient experience. In 2005, Hill Physicians received $5.9 million in funds under the IHA program, but actually distributed $26 million in performance rewards (Hill Physicians, 2005).

---

[1]The Diabetes Physician Recognition Program was developed by the American Diabetes Association and the National Committee for Quality Assurance (NCQA).

[2]The Heart/Stroke Physician Recognition Program was developed by the American Heart Association/American Stroke Association and NCQA.

[3]The Physician Practice Connections was developed by Bridges to Excellence and NCQA.

The Experience of the United Kingdom

Standing in contrast to the pay-for-performance programs in the U.S. commercial insurance market is the recent General Practitioner (GP) contract with Britain's National Health Service (NHS) (Roland, 2004; Smith and York, 2004). The arrangement instituted under this contract awards a substantial portion of compensation according to performance on 146 quality indicators. The program targets physician practices, which generally have fewer than five physicians, rather than individual physicians, and pays according to overall performance using a balanced scorecard (i.e., points are awarded for each of the 146 indicators, and the total score is then used as the basis for payment). In addition to performance bonuses, practices are provided with subsidies for infrastructure improvements, as well as additional staffing. The plan is to put approximately 18 percent of GP income at risk, to be distributed subsequently on the basis of performance measures. Financial penalties for persistent low performance are also planned for future years.

Of note are several important differences between the NHS and Medicare that relate to the ease of implementation and effectiveness of a pay-for-performance program. Every NHS patient must register with an individual practitioner who assumes responsibility for that patient's care. Additionally, the United Kingdom is in the process of instituting a uniform national computerized information system that will include capabilities to automate reporting on the specific measures employed. Most physicians in the United States contract with multiple private and public payers, and many plans with pay-for-performance programs do not account for a large portion of a physician's income. Moreover, the majority of physician award programs in the United States do not put more than 5 percent of compensation at risk (Rosenthal et al., 2004).

Previous programs in the United Kingdom showed positive responses to financial incentives (Smith and York, 2004). A "fundholding experiment" from 1991 to 1998 that gave practitioners fixed budgets for providing secondary care and pharmaceuticals to their patients ultimately resulted in fewer inpatient procedures and reduced patient waiting times. A program in East Kent from 1998 to 2000 defined disease management targets that practitioners had to meet or repay funds. Both of these programs required new money initially; however, the first created incentives for efficiency savings, while the second relied on a reverse withhold to encourage quality improvement.

Common Themes Among Pay-for-Performance Programs

The majority of incentive arrangements target a mix of population-based measures of clinical quality and patient experience measures (Rosenthal et al., 2004). According to a recent survey, payers are also increasingly providing direct incentives for the adoption of information technology and for performance on cost-efficiency metrics (AIS, 2004).

In almost all cases, pay-for-performance sponsors reward all physicians whose performance exceeds an absolute threshold (e.g., at least 80 percent of patients with coronary artery disease undergo appropriate cholesterol screening) or all physicians above a given percentile rank based on the level of performance. Thus, quality improvement is not explicitly required for the receipt of a bonus, and the incentives to improve vary with baseline performance. With an absolute performance threshold, physicians whose baseline performance is high need only maintain the status quo to receive payment. For physicians with the lowest performance, the award may not be sufficient to balance the cost of making the required dramatic improvement.

Most of the early pay-for-performance programs for physicians targeted primary care domains (although payments were often to multispecialty groups). More recently, payers also appear to be measuring and rewarding the quality of care delivered by specialists. According to a private survey, more than two-thirds of current pay-for-performance programs now cover specialists, including cardiologists, obstetrician/gynecologists, orthopedists, gastroenterologists, otolaryngologists, and general surgeons (AIS, 2004).

Pay for Performance in Medicare

While measurement systems have provided an impetus for continuing improvement in the quality of care in the Medicare program, overall change has been slow. To date, CMS has invested heavily in the collection and reporting of data on the quality of care of health plans, hospitals, and other institutional providers. While information-based approaches continue to evolve, reliance on benchmarking, subtle pressure from purchasers, and the market impact of individual patient choice are unlikely to eliminate the gap between optimal, evidence-based medicine and actual practice. However, these efforts do lay the groundwork for an effective pay-for-performance program by generating critical baseline information and the infrastructure that will serve as the base for the reward system.

A broad policy rationale for a Medicare pay-for-performance program is the opportunity to improve not only the overall quality of care for Medicare enrollees, but also the care provided to other populations. Many quality improvement investments involve fixed costs, such as those for information technology or training, whose benefits will accrue to all patients. In addition, the added market power of Medicare will magnify the importance of the existing pay-for-performance programs of health plans and may have further positive spillover effects if other payers follow the lead of CMS in payment reform, as was the case with prospective payment systems.

The objectives of pay for performance are to:

• Encourage the most rapid feasible performance improvement by all providers.
• Support innovation and constructive change throughout the health care system to achieve clinical quality improvements, patient-centered care, and efficient use of health resources.
• Promote better outcomes of care, especially through coordination of care across provider settings and time, especially in the treatment of chronic disease.

Pay for performance is not simply a mechanism to reward those who perform well; rather, its purpose is to encourage redesign and transformation of the health care system to ensure high-quality care for all. In such a system, all participants—providers, purchasers, and beneficiaries—can potentially benefit.

As pay-for-performance programs go forward, it will be crucial to develop a strong learning system within the Medicare enterprise to ensure successful implementation and ongoing improvement (see Chapter 6). The evidence base to support pay for performance is still emerging (see below) and implementation efforts should encompass extensive testing and evaluation to assess the effects of the new system. While pay for performance appears to induce change in some health care environments, it cannot by itself create either the high-performing health care system or the payment reform envisioned in the previous reports of the Institute of Medicine's (IOM's) *Pathways to Quality Health Care* series. Ideally, the contributions of payment reform should be compared with the outcomes that could be produced by other mechanisms, such as continuing medical education, accreditation, and consumer activation, which may also be linked to financial incentives. Such an assessment was beyond the scope of this study. Other nonfinancial mechanisms, such as public reporting, benefit redesign, and professional and public education, are also critical components of a far-reaching quality improvement strategy. All of these efforts should be aligned with pay-for-performance programs in order to ensure a common goal and synergistic effects.

Rewarding Beneficiaries

In designing a pay-for-performance program for Medicare, financial rewards could be directed at providers, beneficiaries, or both. For example, mechanisms could be devised to allow those consumers who improved their lifestyles (to promote better health outcomes) to share with providers in the savings that resulted from the prevention of consequent and more expensive treatments, such as avoidable hospitalizations. Co-pays, deductibles, or premiums could be reduced for those beneficiaries who used designated high-performance providers. However, not all beneficiaries have equal access to those providers deemed high performers, and many hospitals that have excellent reputations for certain medical procedures are not necessarily high performers on all dimensions of quality (Jha and Epstein, 2006). While many possible designs for rewarding beneficiaries could be considered, the evidence base is not yet robust enough to be used to determine how consumer rewards should be structured on a broad level. In interpreting its charge and in an effort to set parameters for what could reasonably and competently be accomplished in Medicare in the short term, the committee did not evaluate beneficiary-oriented approaches, important as they may be. Rather, this report focuses on the provider side of pay for performance.

Pay for Performance and Care Coordination

The deficiencies of the current payment system, as previously described, include its inability to recognize, encourage, or even merely pay for the intentional coordination of patient care across settings and time. The failure to measure these transitions was discussed extensively in the first report in the *Pathways to Quality Health Care* series, *Performance Measurement: Accelerating Improvement* (IOM, 2006b). In the current health care system, care is often fragmented and not well coordinated. The need for measures for use in evaluating, and ultimately rewarding, the coordination of care is necessary to quality improvement with regard to both monitoring gains in clinical quality and reducing inefficiencies. For example, improved coordination of care management could potentially result in a reduction in hospital admissions (Rich et al., 1995; Bodenheimer, 1999; Bodenheimer and Fernandez, 2005). Care coordination measures that might help achieve this end have been developed by Eric Coleman at the University of Colorado (IOM, 2006b). One measure of care coordination in the treatment of congestive heart failure patients is part of CMS's Hospital Compare initiative, although it is not among the first 10 measures that hospitals are being encouraged to report. And the Institute for Healthcare Improvement's 100,000 Lives Campaign includes medication reconciliation for patients being discharged from hospitals (IHI, 2006; Manno and Hayes, 2006). Pay for performance has the potential to act as a catalyst for improved care coordination through program design, making it possible to reward performance based on outcomes by disease, instead of rewarding providers on the basis of individual services at a single point in time. This aspect of pay for performance is elaborated upon further in Chapters 3 through 5.

THE RESEARCH BASE ON PAY FOR PERFORMANCE

The theory behind pay for performance is derived from the basic economic principle that when one pays more for a certain attribute or dimension of a good or service, more of that attribute or dimension is supplied. While this principle tends to hold true in most markets, the introduction of new incentives linked to performance in health care delivery is relatively new. More than 100 pay-for-performance programs have been initiated in the health care arena in the past decade, yet very few studies have assessed their impact empirically (Petersen et al.,2006; Rosenthal and Frank, 2006). Hence, little evidence for the efficacy of pay for performance in the health care setting exists at this time.

Research in the Health Care Sector

In synthesizing the available research literature, the committee identified pay-for-performance studies that demonstrated both positive effects on processes of care (Beaulieu and Horrigan, 2005; Rosenthal et al., 2005b) and negative (but not statistically significant) effects (Beaulieu and Horrigan, 2005). Most studies have failed to demonstrate any significant effects on processes of care (Rosenthal et al., 2005b; Rosenthal and Frank, 2006). However, many of these studies focused on incentives that affected only a small portion of provider income. Early results of experimental projects have also shown that pay for performance can influence positive changes in nontargeted care practices. For example, a physician targeted improvement in immunization rates; as a consequence, documentation of immunizations improved more than the rates themselves (Fairbrother et al., 1999). In general, however, as noted above, a robust literature demonstrating that pay-for-performance strategies lead to improved health outcomes does not yet exist (although this connection may be implicit, as when a measure is evidence-based, such as use of beta-blockers after myocardial infarction). Indeed, one study that examined clinical quality of hospital care for acute myocardial infarction found that performance on process measures accounted for only 6 percent of the variation in 30-day mortality rates (Bradley et al., 2006). The researchers concluded that performance on process measures could not, in this case, reliably predict mortality outcomes. Therefore, the relationship between payment incentives and health outcomes remains uncertain. Overall, however, fewer than 20 studies designed to demonstrate the effectiveness of pay-for-performance programs in improving the quality of care have been conducted (see Appendix B) (Petersen et al., 2006).

The research literature identifies key considerations that require attention when a pay-for-performance program is being designed. Most important is the level of reward necessary to stimulate significant changes in provider behavior or processes of care. In this connection, it must be noted that, as the literature remains silent on how much additional payment is needed to drive change in the domains of clinical quality, patient-centeredness, and efficiency, it is unclear whether a business case can be made for any and all stakeholders in the health care system for pay-for-performance programs. Second is whether financial rewards by themselves can change practice, or other quality improvement initiatives must be implemented as well to achieve positive results (Beaulieu and Horrigan, 2005; Rosenthal et al., 2005b). Third is the issue of designing a system in which low-performing providers can achieve at least the same rate of improvement as high performers. Further experimentation and research are needed to answer these and related questions (Dudley et al., 2004; Rosenthal et al., 2005a, 2005b).

Research in Other Sectors

Outside of the health care sector, a variety of studies of analogous incentive programs have yielded results that may be instructive (Rosenthal and Frank, 2006). Pay for performance has been widely introduced in the education field, and several recent experiments have documented improvements in test scores and other outcomes under these programs (Grumbach et al., 1999; Lavy, 2002). One of these studies also demonstrated that pay for performance was more cost-effective (produced a larger impact for the same expenditure) than direct subsidies for new programs and additional staff time (Lavy, 2002). Pay for performance has also been incorporated into federal contracts for job training programs. Studies examining these programs have found that pay for performance had a positive impact on the rate of job placement and average earnings of trainees, even after accounting for gaming on the part of contractors. Finally, the most commonly observed use of pay for performance is for executive compensation. Corporate executives are frequently awarded performance bonuses based on measures of profitability or market value. According to recent reviews of this extensive literature, results of studies of executive compensation suggest that pay-for-performance programs, typically in the form of stock-based compensation, cause executives to improve firm value (Murphy, 1999; Mishra et al., 2000). It is also worth noting that many observers have raised concern that these types of incentive programs may potentially inhibit beneficial long-term investments that do not provide returns in the short term.

Conclusions

It is difficult to draw conclusions for the health care sector based on the existing evidence on pay for performance. Findings based on observational data are suspect, and suitable natural experiments are lacking. The negative studies in the health care literature used small rewards and incentives based on performance relative to peers, so physicians had no way to know what performance levels would ensure a bonus. Overall, past studies have yielded no clear guidance on the appropriate magnitude of performance-based compensation.

MONITORING FOR UNINTENDED CONSEQUENCES

As noted above, more than 100 pay-for-performance programs have been implemented in the health care sector (Med-Vantage Inc., 2006). These initiatives constitute a rich source of experience regarding the impact of this innovation in health care financing, experience that can help answer questions about what works that are asked by all stakeholders. Concrete data with which to assess the benefits and identify the unintended adverse consequences of the approach are increasingly becoming available; quantification of the impact of pay-for-performance programs is possible, however, only if they are evaluated thoughtfully and systematically. Such evaluation requires careful planning.

Evidence for unintended or unexpected consequences of pay for performance outside of the health care arena, such as gaming in return-to-work and school programs, is relatively well established (Burgess and Ratto, 2003; Courty and Marschke, 2004). In health care, if providers are paid based on performance according to outcome criteria, they may attempt to select healthier patients to maximize net revenues. Other possible negative effects of targeted incentives, such as reductions in various dimensions of quality of care in areas not targeted for financial rewards (which may be a particular concern in primary care because of the broad scope of practice), have not been evaluated empirically. While providers for the most part have the best interests of their patients in mind, such unintended adverse consequences may be a real concern. Table 2-3 is a nonexhaustive listing of some of these potential unintended adverse consequences, each of which is reviewed below. Further experience may identify additional concerns.

Decreased Access

Improved quality of care overall is a highly desirable goal, but it should not be achieved at the expense of decreased access to care. Access to necessary services forms the foundation for high-quality care. A meaningful decrease in access to care resulting from the implementation of a pay-for-performance program constitutes an unacceptable outcome.

In their efforts to reach performance thresholds that will result in augmented payment, providers may exclude patients from their practices who

TABLE 2-3 Potential Unintended Adverse Consequences of Pay for Performance

Decreased Access	Increased Disparities	Marginalized Comprehensive Integrated Care	Impeded Knowledge Transfer and Innovation	Demoralized Workforce	Forestalled Reform Efforts	Shifted Costs
Denial of high-risk or noncompliant patients	Creation of incentives for tiering	Promotion of management to the measure or condition	Decreased sharing of best practices and misadventures	Withdrawal of providers from Medicare	Ignorance of other possible reform efforts	Shift of costs to the private sector
Creation of unmet demand for "successful" providers	Disadvantage to undercapitalized practices	Diversion of resources from nonmeasured areas of care	Slowed uptake of nonmeasured practices	Stalled progress in quality agenda	Stalled progress in quality agenda	Shift of costs to consumers

are known to be at high risk for adverse clinical outcomes. As the evidence base continues to grow, providers will be better able to identify prospectively those patients likely to respond poorly to their care. Process-based performance measures may exert a similar adverse selection pressure. Noncompliant patients constitute a particularly frustrating group of patients to manage, putting health care providers at risk for poor performance based on measures of both process and outcome. If providers react by avoiding these patients to keep their performance scores high, the result could be restricted access to care and worsened health. This is the case especially for the old or chronically ill; initially at higher risk, their health status is more likely to deteriorate and at a faster rate if their access to care is limited. Therefore, researchers must make the investigation of risk adjustment for performance measures a high priority. For example, pay-for-performance programs might be structured to give greater rewards to providers who treat high-risk patients (see Chapter 4). If pay for performance is to realize its full potential for change, it will be necessary to engage providers in the care of these challenging patients.

The public reporting of provider performance may also contribute to decreased access. As emphasized throughout this report, public reporting is a cardinal feature of health care reform as it enhances transparency. It can be a powerful motivator to guide change in provider behavior and provide consumers with key data on which to base good decisions (Shaller et al., 2003). Both of these effects are thought to result in higher-quality health care, which in turn represents better value (Marshall et al., 2000; Mason and Street, 2006). At the same time, however, there is concern that the public reporting of provider performance could have unintended adverse consequences. Health care consumers, both individual patients and payers for health care services, would likely seek out the high-quality providers. Providers shown to perform at lower levels might opt to reduce their Medicare caseloads in favor of participants in private plans. As a result, some consumers could be denied access to the care they desire.

Increased Disparities

Previous IOM reports have highlighted disparities in quality of care that occur along many specific dimensions, including geographic region; provider type; and patient age, sex, and ethnicity (IOM, 2002, 2005). Disparate care is, by definition, low-quality care, and pay for performance could exacerbate such disparities. Populations most affected by disparities in health care are cared for disproportionately by undercapitalized providers who are likely to lack the resources necessary to invest in the infrastructure (such as health information technology) needed to facilitate participation in pay for performance. Nevertheless, the health care services they offer constitute a critical safety net. The same market forces that will operate to improve or eliminate the cohort of providers who perform poorly may leave populations subject to disparities in care with fewer provider options than they had before. Pay-for-performance programs must therefore be carefully designed to identify relationships that exist between populations subject to disparate care and poorly performing providers. Objective assessment will help limit cultural bias in performance measurement.

Marginalized Comprehensive Integrated Care

The application of performance measures in the evaluation of health care for a particular condition (e.g., diabetes mellitus) or preventive service (e.g., breast cancer screening) poses the risk of decreasing performance and thereby compromising the quality of care being provided in areas that are not the focus of pay for performance. Pay for performance could encourage this tendency to manage to the measures, focusing efforts excessively on those measures that yield the greatest financial return. At the same time, however, this could be beneficial by focusing efforts on areas with the greatest need for improvement, such as the treatment of chronic diseases.

Additionally, measures may conflict with one another, ultimately causing harm to patients. This concern reinforces the need, articulated in the *Performance Measurement* report (IOM, 2006b), to develop a comprehensive set of performance measures as rapidly as possible. The present report articulates the need for measures that reward three key domains of care: clinical quality, patient-centeredness, and efficiency. As noted earlier, a single-minded focus on clinical quality can lead to increased health care costs through overuse of services. A similar narrow focus on efficiency could compromise clinical quality and raise at least the appearance of a fundamental conflict of interest. And performance measures that place undue emphasis on clinical quality or efficiency are unlikely to be patient-centered.

A comprehensive portfolio of performance measures must reflect consensus around the vision of a reformed and integrated health care system designed to achieve the goals articulated in the *Quality Chasm* report (IOM, 2001). For example, prompt, understandable, and empathetic communication to the patient of the results of a magnetic resonance scan is as important as the technical quality and value of the imaging study itself; ideally, financial incentives should be restructured, based on valid and robust measures of performance, to encourage both.

Impeded Knowledge Transfer and Innovation

In the health care sector, best practices are adopted at a surprisingly and disconcertingly slow rate (Lomas et al., 1993; Bates et al., 2003). While health care presents a unique set of challenges for practice improvement, innovations that are evidence based and have been demonstrated to improve the quality of care can take in excess of 17 years to become common practice (Balas and Boren, 2000). Delay in the development or implementation of best practices has substantial human and financial costs. Open dissemination of experience is necessary to harness the capacity of the health care industry to improve. Pay-for-performance programs could unintentionally subordinate collaboration to competition. Providers following a more economically directed model of care might hesitate to share successful practice improvement strategies with their competitors, fearing that doing so would put at risk not only the financial incentives offered through pay for performance, but also the competitive advantage that these successful innovations would offer in negotiating with patients and insurers.

It is difficult to know how best to prevent this from occurring. Clearly the business case for cooperation must be made as solidly and quickly as possible so that providers will be motivated to share both successful strategies and barriers to implementation they may identify. Government is limited in its ability to bring about this type of interchange. Entities such as Medicare's Quality Improvement Organizations might provide a forum for exchange of such information, fostering the creation of a culture of quality improvement (IOM, 2006a).

A separate compelling concern is that pay for performance could inadvertently stifle long-term innovation by shifting the focus of quality improvement exclusively to the achievement of short-term goals. While it is important to reward interventions that result in short-term improvements, it is essential as well not to suppress the experimentation and innovation that can lead to new procedures, applications, and approaches that can generate long-term continuous improvement in quality. Successful pay-for-performance programs must not foster the development of a new status quo that is better, but incomplete.

Demoralized Workforce

Pay for performance must be structured to promote higher-quality care and cost control, but not at the expense of driving providers from the health care arena. Provider acceptance will be a large point of contention in any pay-for-performance initiative. If payment under such a program is perceived by providers as unfair, they may become increasingly demoralized. Additionally, if the burden on providers of participating in a Medicare pay-for-performance program is too overwhelming (relative to the potential rewards), providers may withdraw from participation in Medicare, causing serious access issues in some geographic regions in addition to those discussed above. For example, fewer physicians are choosing primary care as their field, in part because of lower income and increased workload (Moore and Showstack, 2003). An even further decrease in payments could exacerbate this problem. The problem may be compounded if decreased payments lead those already in primary care practices to leave the profession (Sox, 2003). Lack of acceptance may increase if providers are not consulted during the process of program implementation in order to allay some of these concerns.

The committee concludes that most providers have the capacity and desire to improve the care they deliver—an essential component of a successful pay-for-performance program. A lack of acceptance by providers would not only disrupt the management of a pay-for-performance program, but potentially hinder the entire quality agenda. If payers rely on pay for performance as a pathway to improving care and health outcomes, progress along that pathway will be forestalled if a majority of providers refuse to participate. Fundamentally, providers must believe in and accept the system not just because of the rewards they may receive, but also because they believe in its ability to advance the quality agenda. That goal will not be realized if action to achieve the system is delayed by a lack of acceptance of program terms among providers.

Forestalled Reform Efforts

If payers or policy makers focus too intensely on pay for performance as a major solution to the current inadequacies of the payment system, they may fail to recognize other mechanisms that might work as well or better. In the context of the need for pay for performance to be a learning system, as emphasized throughout this report, payers and policy makers should remain aware of other options that could enhance or replace pay-for-performance strategies. On the other hand, policy makers could decelerate progress by focusing too much on potential unintended negative consequences, diverting attention from the intended positive consequences of rewarding higher quality and better outcomes to improve the quality of care received by all Medicare beneficiaries. This is not meant to imply that the implementation of pay for performance should proceed without caution, but to emphasize that the possible unintended adverse consequences should not hinder progress.

Shifted Costs

Assuming the pay-for-performance program will involve a reduction in base payments (see Chapter 3 on use of existing funds), when Medicare pays less for a service, providers could try to shift those unreimbursed costs to the private sector. Cost shifting results when decreased reimbursements by one payer leads providers (by force of market power) to demand higher rates of payment from another payer (Lee et al., 2003). For example, researchers examining data from the late 1980s through the early 1990s found that lower Medicare payments to hospitals were associated with statistically significant increases in payment rates to hospitals by private payers (Zwanziger et al., 2000). As a result, the burden of some costs may eventually shift directly to the consumer (Gabel et al., 2002; Lee and Tollen, 2002). For example, increased costs to private payers may lead to increased premiums and copays for the consumer, which in turn could contribute to other potential adverse consequences already described, such as decreased access. Thus decreased payments might save costs for Medicare, but lead to an undue burden for private payers and consumers. However, if the main private payers were to follow Medicare's lead on pay for performance, the opportunity for such cost shifting would be reduced.

Conclusions

Quality improvement is a continuous and dynamic process; caution in the design of pay-for-performance programs is necessary to ensure that successful programs do not foster the development of a new status quo—one that is better, but incomplete. Overall, any pay-for-performance program must be designed as a learning system that will allow for modifications in response to feedback obtained, including unintended positive consequences. Additionally, the program must incorporate mechanisms designed to monitor for unintended negative consequences and allow for rapid correction to prevent any resulting harm. These issues are discussed in more detail in Chapter 6.

A FIRST STEP TOWARD PAYMENT SYSTEM REFORM

The many pay-for-performance programs now planned or in place have been supported with considerable resources and enthusiastic commitment over a remarkably short period of time. Many public policy makers share the enthusiasm of their colleagues in the private sector, and state and federal programs are poised to follow the lead of private insurers. Unfortunately, clear goals, the best intentions, and a substantial investment of human and financial capital do not guarantee success in the implementation of a pay-for-performance program.

The urgency of the quality problem in the environment of the current payment system demands that steps be taken now to align payment with the six quality aims of the *Quality Chasm* report (IOM, 2001) and improve health outcomes. The committee recognizes that no perfect payment strategy has yet been identified to advance these goals. However, the economic rationale behind and early experience with pay for performance suggests that it offers an initial and interim pathway to change, although more fundamental restructuring of the payment system may be necessary in the future. Therefore, the committee makes the following recommendation:

> **Recommendation 1: The Secretary of the Department of Health and Human Services (DHHS) should implement pay for performance in Medicare using a phased approach as a stimulus to foster comprehensive and systemwide improvements in the quality of health care.**

The committee concludes that as pay for performance is implemented, the aim should be to move toward rewarding comprehensive care as soon as possible, instead of focusing payments and rewards on individual episodes of care in isolated settings. In this sense, the committee envisions that as pay for performance evolves, shifts should occur from rewarding process measures toward rewarding outcome measures, and from rewarding by setting toward rewarding by health condition. Initial pay-for-performance programs will be limited by the availability of reliable measures and the structure of the current payment system. Therefore, for example, while the availability and reliability of measures may necessitate an initial focus on rewarding process more than outcome measures and rewarding by setting instead of by condition, the committee foresees this balance shifting over time. It will be important to use research and evaluation techniques to identify milestones by which this shift should be encouraged. The details of a phased implementation are discussed in more detail in Chapter 5.

SUMMARY

This chapter has examined the promise of pay for performance as a lever in the redesign of the current health care payment system. The current system does not reward high-quality care, nor does it provide incentives for providers to improve their performance in care delivery. Medicare expenditures have continued to grow rapidly, while improvements in the overall quality of care have not kept pace. Pay for performance holds promise as one component of a redesigned approach to create incentives for improving the quality of care. Many pay-for-performance initiatives have been undertaken in both the public and private sectors, offering some initial feedback, but a larger effort is needed to create changes on the scale necessary to improve the nation's health care system. Medicare wields sufficient power to act as a leader in this effort. While pay for performance appears to hold much promise, the committee cautions that it alone cannot reform the health care system. Additionally, a pay-for-performance program of this scale must be an evolving learning system that can adapt to knowledge gained and monitor for unintended negative consequences. The following chapters describe how pay for performance in Medicare could be designed. Chapter 3 addresses funding alternatives, Chapter 4 issues surrounding the distribution of those funds, and Chapter 5 specific details of program implementation.

REFERENCES

AIS. 2004. *Case Studies in Health Plan Pay-for-Performance Program.* Washington, DC: Atlantic Information Services, Inc.

Balas EA, Boren SA. 2000. Managing clinical knowledge for health care improvement. *Yearbook of Medical Informatics 2000: Patient-Centered Systems.* Stuttgart: Schattaver Verlasgesellschaft. Pp. 65–70.

Bates DW, Kuperman GJ, Wang S, Gandhi T, Kittler A, Volk L, Spurr C, Khorasani R, Tanasijevic M, Middleton B. 2003. Ten commandments for effective clinical decision support: Making the practice of evidence-based medicine a reality. *Journal of Medical Informatics Association* 10(6):523–530.

Beaulieu ND, Horrigan DR. 2005. Putting smart money to work for quality improvement. 40(5 I):1318–1334.

Bodenheimer T. 1999. Disease management—Promises and pitfalls. *New England Journal of Medicine* 340(15):1202–1205.

Bodenheimer T, Fernandez A. 2005. High and rising health care costs. Part 4: Can costs be controlled while preserving quality? *Annals of Internal Medicine* 143(1):26–31.

Bradley EH, Herrin J, Elbel B, McNamara RL, Magid DJ, Nallamothu BK, Wang Y, Normand S-LT, Spertus, JA, Krumholz HZ. 2006. Hospital quality for acute myocardial infarction: Correlation among process measures and relationship with short-term mortality. *Journal of the American Medical Association* 296(1):72–78.

Burgess S, Ratto M. 2003. The role of incentives in the public sector: Issues and evidence. *Oxford Review of Economic Policy* 19(2):285–300.

CMS (Centers for Medicare and Medicaid Services). 2006a. *National Health Expenditures by Type of Service and Source of Funds.* [Online]. Available: http://www.cms.hhs.gov/NationalHealthExpendData/02_NationalHealthAccountsHistorical.asp#TopofPage [accessed April, 18, 2006].

CMS. 2006b. *Rewarding Superior Quality Care: The Premier Hospital Quality Incentive Demonstration.* [Online]. Available: http://www.cms.hhs.gov/HospitalQualityInits/downloads/HospitalPremierFS200602.pdf [accessed June 9, 2006].

CMS. 2006c. *Prospective Payment Systems—General Information.* [Online]. Available: http://www.cms.hhs.gov/ProspMedicareFeeSvcPmtGen/ [accessed May 31, 2006].

Cohen JW, Spector WD. 1996. The effect of Medicaid reimbursement on quality of care in nursing homes. *Journal of Health Economics* 15(1):23–48.

Courty P, Marschke G. 2004. An empirical investigation of gaming responses to explicit performance incentives. *Journal of Labor Economics* 22(1):23–56.

Dudley R, Frolich A, Robinowitz DL, Talavera JA, Broadhead P, Luft HS. 2004. *Strategies to Support Quality-Based Purchasing: A Review of the Evidence.* Rockville, MD: Agency for Healthcare Research and Quality.

Fairbrother G, Hanson KL, Friedman S, Butts GC. 1999. The impact of physician bonuses, enhanced fees, and feedback on childhood immunization coverage rates. *American Journal of Public Health* 89(2):171–175.

Gabel J, Levitt L, Holve E, Pickreigh J, Whitmore H, Dhont K, Hawkins S, Rowland D. 2002. Job-based health benefits in 2002: Some important trends. *Health Affairs* 21(5): 143–151.

Ginsburg PB, Grossman JM. 2005. When the price isn't right: How inadvertent payment incentives drive medical care. *Health Affairs* w5.376.

Grumbach K, Selby JV, Damberg C, Bindman AB, Quesenberry C Jr., Truman A, Uratsu C. 1999. Resolving the gatekeeper conundrum: What patients value in primary care and referrals to specialists. *Journal of the American Medical Association* 282(3):261–266.

Hill Physicians. 2005. *Hill Physicians Medical Group: 2005 Annual Report*. [Online]. Available: http://www.hillphysicians.com/HPMG_AR2005.pdf [accessed August 3, 2006].

Hodgkin D, McGuire TG. 1994. Payment levels and hospital response to prospective payment. *Journal of Health Economics* 13(1):1–29.

IHA (Integrated Healthcare Association). 2006a. *IHA News Release*. [Online]. Available: http://www.iha.org/020606.htm [accessed August 3, 2006].

IHA. 2006b. *IHA P4P Measurement Set*. [Online]. Available: http://www.iha.org/p4pyr4/fmy4.pdf [accessed August 3, 2006].

IHI (Institute for Healthcare Improvement). 2006. *Getting Started Kit: Prevent Adverse Drug Events (Medication Reconciliation)*. [Online]. Available: http://www.ihi.org/NR/rdonlyres/47D5AE1C-0B29-4A59-8D58-BABF8F4E829F/0/ADEHowtoGuideFINAL5_25.pdf [accessed June 8, 2006].

IOM (Institute of Medicine). 2001. *Crossing the Quality Chasm: A New Health System for the 21st Century*. Washington, DC: National Academy Press.

IOM 2002. *Insuring Health—Care Without Coverage: Too Little, Too Late*. Committee on the Consequences of Uninsurance, eds. Washington, DC: The National Academies Press.

IOM. 2005. *Quality Through Collaboration: The Future of Rural Health*. Washington, DC: The National Academies Press.

IOM 2006a. *Medicare's Quality Improvement Organization Program: Maximizing Potential*. Washington, DC: The National Academies Press.

IOM. 2006b. *Performance Measurement: Accelerating Improvement*. Washington, DC: The National Academies Press.

Jha AK, Epstein AM. 2006. The predictive accuracy of the New York state coronary artery bypass surgery report-card system. *Health Affairs* 25(3):844–855.

Kaiser Family Foundation. 2005. *Medicare Advantage Fact Sheet*. Washington, DC: Henry J. Kaiser Family Foundation.

Kautter J, Pope GC, Trisolini M, Bapat B, Olmsted E, and Klosterman M. 2004. *Physician Group Practice Demonstration Bonus Methodology Specifications*. Unpublished.

Landro L. 2004, September 17. Booster shot: To get doctors to do better, health plans try cash bonuses. *The Wall Street Journal*.

Lavy V. 2002. Evaluating the effect of teachers' group performance incentives on pupil achievement. *Journal of Political Economy* 110(6):1286–1317.

Lee JS, Tollen L. 2002. How low can you go? The impact of reduced benefits and increased cost sharing. *Health Affairs* w290–241.

Lee JS, Berenson RA, Mayes R, Gauthier AK. 2003. Medicare payment policy: Does cost shifting matter? *Health Affairs* w3, 480–488.

Lomas J, Sisk JE, Stocking B. 1993. From evidence to practice in the United States, the United Kingdom, and Canada. *The Milbank Quarterly* 71(3):405–410.

Manno MS, Hayes DD. 2006. Best-practice interventions: How medication reconciliation saves lives. *Nursing* 36(3):63–64.

Marshall MN, Shekelle PG, Leatherman S, Brook RH. 2000. The release of performance data: What do we expect to gain? A review of the evidence. *Journal of the American Medical Association* 283(14):1866–1874.

Mason A, Street A. 2006. Publishing outcome data: Is it an effective approach? *Journal of Evaluation in Clinical Practice* 12(1):37–48.

Med-Vantage Inc. 2006. *Pay for Performance.* [Online]. Available: http://medvantageinc.com/Content/solutions.p4p.php4 [accessed June 9, 2006].

MedPAC (Medicare Payment Advisory Commission). 2005. *MedPAC Data Runs.* Washington, DC: MedPAC.

MedPAC. 2006. *Report to the Congress: Medicare Payment Policy.* Washington, DC: MedPAC.

Mishra CS, McConaughy DL, Gobeli DH. 2000. Effectiveness of CEO pay-for-performance. *Review of Financial Economics* 9(1):1–13.

Moore G, Showstack JA. 2003. Primary care medicine in crisis: Toward reconstruction and renewal. *Annals of Internal Medicine* 138(3):244–247.

Murphy K. 1999. *Executive Compensation. Handbook of Labor Economics.* New York: Elsevier Science Pub. Co.

PBGH (Pacific Business Group on Health). 2005. *Aligning Physician Incentives: Lessons and Perspectives from California.* [Online]. Available: http://www.pbgh.org/programs/documents/PhysIncentivesReport_09-01-05final.pdf [accessed August 2, 2006].

Petersen LA, Woodard LD, Urech T, Daw C, Sookanan S. 2006. Does pay-for-performance improve the quality of health care? *Annals of Internal Medicine* 145(4):265–272.

Premier Inc. 2006. *HQI Demonstration.* [Online]. Available: http://www.premierinc.com/all/quality/hqi/ [accessed June 9, 2006].

Remus D. December 2005. *Pay for Performance—CMS/Premier Hospital Quality Incentive Demonstration Project (Year 1 Results).* [Online]. Available: http://www.premierinc.com/all/quality/hqi/results/year-1-results-participant-calll.pdf [accessed June 9, 2006].

Rich MW, Beckham V, Wittenberg C, Leven CL, Freedland KE, Carney RM. 1995. A multidisciplinary intervention to prevent the readmission of elderly patients with congestive heart failure. *New England Journal of Meddicine* 333(18):1190–1195.

Robinson JC. 2001. Theory and practice in the design of physician payment incentives. *The Milbank Quarterly* 79(2):149–177.

Roland M. 2004. Linking physicians' pay to the quality of care: A major experiment in the United Kingdon. *New England Journal of Medicine* 351(14):1448–1454.

Rosenthal MB, Frank RG. 2006. What is the empirical basis for paying for quality in health care? *Medical Care Research and Review* 63(2):135–157.

Rosenthal MB, Fernandopulle R, Song HR, Landon B. 2004. Paying for quality: Providers' incentives for quality improvement. *Health Affairs* 23(2):127–141.

Rosenthal M, Hsuan C, Milstein A. 2005a. A report card on the freshman class of consumer-directed health plans. *Health Affairs* 24(6):1592–1600.

Rosenthal MB, Frank RG, Li Z, Epstein AM. 2005b. Early experience with pay-for-performance: From concept to practice. *Journal of the American Medical Association* 294(14):1788–1793.

Shaller D, Sofaer S, Findlay SD, Hibbard JH, Delbanco S. 2003. Perspective: Consumers and quality-driven health care: A call to action. *Health Affairs* 22(2):95–101.

Shen J, Andersen R, Brook R, Kominski G, Albert PS, Wenger N. 2004. The effects of payment method on clinical decision-making: Physician responses to clinical scenarios. *Medical Care* 42(3):297–302.

Smith PC, York N. 2004. Quality incentives: The case of U.K. general practitioners—An ambitious U.K. quality improvement initiative offers the potential for enormous gains in the quality of primary health care. *Health Affairs* 23(3):112–118.

Sox HC. 2003. The future of primary care. *Annals of Internal Medicine* 138(3):230–232.

SUNY. May 2001. *Fact Sheet: Medicare Basics.* [Online]. Available: http://www.canton.edu/can/can_start.taf?page=ota_medicare_facts [accessed May 31, 2006].

U.S. GAO (United States Government Accountability Office). 2005. *Medicare Physician Payments: Considerations for Reforming the Sustainable Growth Rate System.* Washington, DC: U.S. Government Printing Office.

White C. 2003. Rehabilitation therapy in skilled nursing facilities: Effects of Medicare's new prospective payment system. *Health Affairs* 22(3):214–223.

Zwanziger J, Melnick GA, Bamezai A. 2000. Can cost shifting continue in a price competitive environment? *Health Economics* 9(3):211–225.

3

Alternative Funding Sources

CHAPTER SUMMARY

Several possible funding sources can be tapped to generate the resources needed for a Medicare pay-for-performance initiative. This chapter examines the process of choosing initial funding sources, including the strengths and weaknesses of each source as a strategy for moving toward a sustainable payment system that rewards care characterized by high clinical quality, patient-centeredness, and efficiency. For each option, the committee considered several important criteria: the adequacy of the source, its stability or reliability, the extent to which different types of providers would consider it to be fair, and the impact of the mechanism on the overall quality of care and health care spending.

While this chapter focuses explicitly on sources of funding, the analysis of these options is unavoidably intertwined with distribution and implementation issues (such as whether reward pools are to be divided by provider setting or aggregated into one large pool). These issues are noted where appropriate; however, more detailed discussion of distribution and implementation is presented in Chapters 4 and 5.

The establishment of a funding pool for any pay-for-performance program has major policy implications. Because funds must be available before any reward payments can be made, creation of a funding pool signals the start of the pay-for-performance program and will send a strong message that the overall quality of care, in addition to the events of care, is about to acquire importance in the payment system. Resistance to any pay-for-performance program is likely to start when the funding sources (the Medicare Trust Funds, purchasers, providers) become apparent. Therefore, decisions about the source(s) require careful consideration of several major design questions. For example, will there be one large reward pool or a separate pool for each provider setting? What pool size will be needed to support rewards of sufficient magnitude to motivate various types of providers? If there is one large pool, what is to be done with those who, because of inadequate performance measures, cannot initially qualify for rewards? While many of these matters are discussed in Chapters 4 and 5, which focus on the distribution of funds and implementation issues, respectively, these questions must be considered when basic decisions on the initial funding source(s) for the rewards are made since all subsequent program decisions will hinge on those choices.

BASIC FUNDING MODELS

The resources needed to support a pay-for-performance program can be obtained from existing funds, from generated savings, or from direct investment (new money). *Existing funds* are monies that are already part of the payment system. This model reduces payments to all or selected types of providers for redistribution to those exhibiting higher quality in examined areas. The reward pool that is divided among those providers who reach specified quality goals may be created by reducing planned fee schedule increases (referred to as "shaving the update"), by withholding a portion of the base payment, or by enacting an explicit set of Medicare program cuts. The *generated-savings* model creates a reward pool from the money saved as a result of the adoption of cost-reducing reforms and efficiencies associated with the effort to improve quality. The *direct-investment* model adds new money from either Medicare's Hospital Insurance trust fund or general revenues and distributes it as bonuses over and above a scheduled payment. Variations on each of these funding sources are discussed in more detail later in this chapter. Although these models represent three distinct approaches to funding, mixed approaches are also possible.

The decision as to the source of funding is important for several reasons. Most important, there will be concern over whether the program is budget neutral—that is, whether it will add to government spending. In an era of high and escalating budget deficits, lawmakers are likely to object to spending more on a program that is already very costly, with expenditures growing rapidly. Provider groups, on the other hand, will want new funds to be used, arguing that payment rates are already too low and that redistributing a portion of these inadequate amounts will leave some with insufficient resources to do their jobs well and respond to new demands. In addition, some types of providers who are adversely affected by the funding mechanism selected will initially not have the opportunity to receive performance rewards. For example, performance measures are insufficiently developed for some specialties and provider types to allow for participation in a pay-for-performance program. This disconnect will cause understandable dissension. Overall, defining the mechanism for the creation of an initial funding pool for a pay-for-performance program is likely to have very real and contentious policy implications.

Models in the Private Sector

The pay-for-performance programs that have emerged in the private sector are frequently characterized as new-money models, whereby providers are paid a bonus on top of the regular fee schedule. However, some of these programs anticipate that the use of performance measures and the bonus structure will generate savings through improved efficiency, as well as long-term savings due to increased use of preventive services. For example, the Bridges to Excellence program invested money up front for bonuses using actuarial models (de Brantes et al., 2003). Box 3-1 describes how the Bridges to Excellence program predetermined an adequate reward pool encompassing both new initial funds and generated savings. The program expected to devote 50 percent of anticipated savings to the reward pool, with the other 50 percent being considered a return on investment to the purchasers.

Other private-sector models include the Integrated Healthcare Association program in California, which rewards physician groups on the basis of clinical performance, patient experience, and use of information technology. Anthem Blue Cross and Blue Shield of New Hampshire pays bonuses to physician groups based on their provision of preventive services, thus making this a prospective generated-savings model.

Some providers are skeptical of these strategies, asserting that the bonuses are financed by redirecting full payment updates rather than by providing new money (Bailit Health Purchasing LLC, 2002). Other bonus programs, including Blue Cross Blue Shield of Massachusetts and Harvard Pilgrim Health Care, generate revenues from a percentage of an annual withhold (Rosenthal et al., 2004). According to stakeholder testimony and a longitudinal study performed by ViPS and Med-Vantage from 2003 through 2005, provider groups favor strategies that generate new and increased income to providers, while purchasers favor budget-neutral approaches (ACHP, 2004, 2005; AAFP, 2005; ACOG, 2005; ACP, 2005; AMA, 2005; Baker and Carter, 2005).

Models in the Public Sector

As discussed in Chapter 2, the Centers for Medicare and Medicaid Services (CMS) has undertaken several pay-for-performance initiatives for multiple provider settings. Because the Office of Management and Budget, in general, insists that demonstrations be budget neutral overall, these initiatives are funded largely on the basis of anticipated savings attributable to

---

BOX 3-1 Bridges to Excellence: Combination of an Adequate Reward Pool and Generated Savings

The Bridges to Excellence program was developed by a coalition of providers, health plans, and employers that worked with General Electric to apply that organization's quality improvement methodology, six sigma, to the health care field (de Brantes et al., 2003). The program's mission included rewarding providers for clinical quality performance. In the initial stages of program development, the coalition identified attributes that would define the needs of providers, consumers, and purchasers. The coalition recognized in particular the need to identify what level of funding would be sufficient to motivate providers to change their behaviors and accept the program (Personal communication, F. de Brantes and R. Galvin, General Electric, January 30, 2006). Within a generated-savings model, actuarial studies were done to quantify generated savings.

Providers participated in focus groups held to determine the levels and types of incentives that would be necessary to motivate change. Other studies on incentive programs were also considered (Bailit Health Purchasing LLC, 2002). Thus the Bridges to Excellence program is an example of how a funding pool for incentives based on the needs of providers was predetermined. The program may also be viewed as having elements of the direct-investment and generated-savings models in that theoretically, new money was put into the program to work on quality improvement in specific areas, and the program expected to reinvest savings into the reward pool.

SOURCE: Personal communication, F. de Brantes and R. Galvin, General Electric, January 30, 2006.

---

improved efficiency. However, most of these initiatives received some new funds to initiate their implementation.

The Experience of the United Kingdom

As described in Chapter 2, the National Health System in the United Kingdom initiated a pay-for-performance program for general health in April 2004. The program links a major portion of payment to performance on clinical indicators, organizational indicators, and patient experience. The British government invested more than $1.8 billion—a more than 20 percent increase over the previous health budget—in new money for bonuses for general practice (Roland, 2004). Previous incentive programs in the United Kingdom had demonstrated positive responses to financial incentives. A "fund holding experiment" from 1991 to 1998 gave practitioners fixed budgets to provide secondary care and pharmaceuticals to their patients; this program ultimately resulted in fewer inpatient procedures and reduced patient waiting times (Smith and York, 2004). A program in East Kent from 1998 to 2000 established disease management targets and required that practitioners repay funds if those targets were not met (Smith and York, 2004). These two initiatives required new money initially; however, the first created incentives for efficiency, which generated savings, while the second relied on a reverse withhold to encourage quality improvement.

GUIDING PRINCIPLES FOR SELECTION OF A FUNDING SOURCE

Evaluation Criteria

The committee considered four criteria when evaluating the merits of alternative funding sources for pay for performance in Medicare: adequacy, stability, fairness, and impact (see Table 3-1).

Adequacy refers to the ability to generate a pool of sufficient size to support (on an ongoing basis) bonuses that are large enough to create meaningful incentives for improved performance. *Stability* refers to the predictability of the source. Will it depend on the annual appropriation decisions of Congress, and therefore be subject to political fluctuations and broader budgetary concerns? Will the size of the pool vary with fluctuations in the strength of the economy? *Fairness* involves the balance between those who are asked to contribute to the reward pool and those who have an opportunity to receive bonuses. This concern relates directly to providers or settings whose payments might be reduced to fund a reward pool but for whom good performance measures do not currently exist, such as specialists, rehabilitation facilities, and long-term care hospitals. Finally, *impact* is related to how each option might affect the Medicare program and its beneficiaries positively or negatively. To what extent might the funding mechanism in

TABLE 3-1 Criteria for Evaluating Alternative Funding Sources

Adequacy	Stability	Fairness	Impact
• Size • Length of time to establish • Ability to influence behavior	• Predictability of source • Sustainability • Complexity of implementation	• Winners and losers • Ability to participate	• Effect on program savings • Effect on quality of care

and of itself encourage efficiency or undermine the quality of care provided to beneficiaries?

Other Considerations

Other factors considered by the committee include the likelihood of stakeholder acceptance of each alternative, its administrative complexity, and its budgetary impact. The committee assigned significant weight to this last dimension, favoring funding approaches that would be budget conscious or, preferably, budget neutral. Budget-neutral approaches are those that do not initially lead to an increase in overall government spending (exclusive of administrative costs). The committee recognizes that there will be added expenses at the provider level associated with data collection and reporting or the implementation of process redesign. The committee agreed that if a funding alternative could not be budget neutral initially, it should at least be budget conscious, ensuring that budget concerns are explicitly recognized and addressed.

Scope

When one is considering how best to fund a pay-for-performance program, overarching decisions must be made concerning the scope of the reward pool. Separate pools could be created for each provider setting, or one aggregate pool could fund rewards for all provider types. The pool could be national or regional in scope. The program could also start with regional pools that were specific to provider types and move over time to a single national pool. However, the creation of regional pools could be too complex from an administrative standpoint and lead to variations in treatment across regions and types of providers that some would consider inequitable. Moreover, multiple pools could undermine efforts to encourage care coordination and lead some categories of providers to attempt to avoid participation altogether.

SHORT-TERM MODELS

In evaluating alternative funding sources for pay for performance, the committee was cautious, realizing that there is no strong evidence base to guide its recommendations. Ideally, CMS would mount a series of staged demonstrations in selected regions of the country, encompassing a well-structured evaluative component, which would allow for systematic evaluation of the effectiveness of different approaches. However, sensing the urgent need for reform, the number of years such demonstrations would take, and the opposition the demonstrations might generate in affected regions, the committee concluded that it would be best to move forward with both short- and long-term strategies. For the short term, the committee considered the three basic models noted above:

- Use of existing funds—pool formed from money already in the health care system.
- Generated savings—pool based on savings (relative to projected spending).
- Direct investment—introduction of new money to work on specific conditions.

Use of Existing Funds

Models based on the use of existing funds create an initial reward pool from the current funding base. Hence, funding of a pay-for-performance program is budget neutral from the start. This type of pool could be created by:

- Using a portion (or all) of scheduled payment updates (known as "shaving the update").
- Reducing base payments by a certain percentage.
- Having Congress establish a reward pool of a predetermined size, spending for which would be offset by enacting a package of specific cuts in the Medicare program that might or might not affect payment rates.

Prominent physician groups in particular have expressed concern about approaches that are budget neutral or provide no new money to fund pay for performance because they are aware that under the sustainable growth rate (SGR) mechanism, physician fees are already scheduled to decline significantly over the next few years, which makes reductions in existing payment rates especially concerning for this provider group (ACHP, 2004, 2005; AAFP, 2005; ACOG, 2005; ACP, 2005; AMA, 2005). An initial reward pool based on shaving the update might be generated from a tax or assessment that reduced the size of the annual update of Medicare payment to providers by one or two percentage points. Alternatively, base payment rates could be reduced by a percentage point or two. The total pool would be paid out annually.

Adequacy

If the updates were shaved or the base payment rate reduced only in the first year, the size of the reward pool would amount to only 1 or 2 percentage points of payments year after year. Substantial uncertainty exists as to whether a pool created by a one-time shaving of the update or a single reduction in the base payment of such a small magnitude would be sufficient to motivate the desired behavioral changes among all types of providers. While institutional providers, such as hospitals, might be motivated by relatively small bonuses, it is doubtful that rewards of one or two percentage points of base payments would be sufficient to motivate physicians to adopt the infrastructure supports, such as data registries, needed to track and monitor patients with chronic conditions so as to ensure that evidence-based care is being delivered.

Initial experience in the private sector suggests that reward thresholds are within the range of 5–15 percent of earnings for physicians and 1–2 percent of gross revenues for hospitals (Personal communication, F. de Brantes and R. Galvin, General Electric, January 30, 2006) (Baker and Carter, 2005; Nussbaum, 2005). Box 3-1, presented earlier, describes how Bridges to Excellence determined an adequate funding pool.

To provide a rough estimate of what this would mean in the Medicare setting, the committee consulted with MedPAC to perform data runs on the total payments that are associated with the three conditions for which a majority of Medicare payments are made—chronic heart failure, coronary artery disease, and diabetes (see Appendix D). To determine the average reward per unique physician identification number (UPIN), the committee made the following assumptions: (1) one-quarter of physicians would not be eligible based on the lack of available adequate measures, (2) only half of physicians would achieve the level of performance required to receive rewards, and (3) 2 percent would be taken from base payments. This results in a denominator of 75,000 physicians receiving rewards. To calculate the numerator, the committee took 2 percent of the total physician fee schedule payments made by Medicare for services associated with treatment of the above-named conditions, or about $6.61 million. Dividing numerator by denominator results in rewards approximating $88 per physician per year (see Table 3-2). While there are other important variables to consider, and this example only uses three conditions, the committee used this calculation to demonstrate that either adding new money or putting a larger proportion of the base payment at risk may be necessary to motivate providers adequately.

The updates or base payments could be reduced by an additional 1 or 2 percentage points in each of the first few years. If this were repeated for each of the first 5 years, the pool available for bonuses would grow gradually, reaching between 5 and 10 percent of baseline base payments by year 5. This pool would support bonuses of 10 to 20 percent of base payments for the top-performing half of physicians.

TABLE 3-2   Example of Rewards per Eligible UPIN
Based on Percentage of Total Payments

Percentage of Payment	Rewards in Dollars per Eligible UPIN (based on total fee schedule payments)
1	44.08
2	88.17
10	440.85
15	661.20

NOTE: Total physician fee schedule payments = $330,627,588.35; UPINs in above examples = 75,000. Numbers are based on services associated with treatment of chronic heart failure, coronary artery disease, and diabetes.

Stability

This option is a budget-neutral strategy that requires no new money and is fiscally prudent in an environment of scarce resources. It could be implemented immediately. The variant of this option that involves shaving the updates is more complex and uncertain than the variant that relies on reducing base payments because not all provider types receive an automatic update, and Congress often reduces the updates called for under law for budgetary or other reasons. In fact, the SGR currently calls for the physicians' fee schedule to undergo negative updates of more than 4 percent annually from 2007 to 2011 (MedPAC, 2006). Approaches based on the use of existing funds are less complex than those based on generated savings because they do not depend on uncertain actuarial estimates of savings generated by policy changes.

Fairness

A major disadvantage of the existing-funds model initially is the likelihood that some providers who would have their payments reduced to generate the reward pool would be unable to compete for bonuses. For example, an across-the-board reduction in the update or the base payments for physicians would affect all physicians, whereas certain specialists or others for whom accurate and reliable performance measures do not yet exist would be precluded from participating initially in a pay-for-performance program. This problem would be compounded among physicians who might face unrecoverable cuts in payment while concurrently facing a negative update. Many would regard this to be unfair, even if it would be a transitional situation. On the other hand, this inequity could create incentives for providers lacking measures to develop them more quickly to become eligible for rewards. If the reward pool were generated from an explicit set of Medicare cuts that did not include reductions in payment rates or updates, however, the program might be more palatable to providers.

Impact

The existing-funds model could have several undesirable impacts. First, cutting payment rates could leave some providers who already had negative Medicare margins with insufficient resources to maintain their current quality of care. Second, some might feel that Medicare rates had become insufficient and thus be less willing to see Medicare beneficiaries, creating access problems. Finally, in an effort to maintain revenues in the face of lower payment rates, providers might increase their rate of services, leading to more low-value or unnecessary care.

Generated Savings

Another budget-neutral approach is to build the reward pool solely from savings generated by efficiencies providers adopt in attempting to improve the overall quality of the care they deliver. Under this model, if spending grows at a slower pace than was projected, the difference between projected and actual spending is made available for performance-based awards. This approach depends on reliable projections of baseline Medicare spending; in the past, such projections have been difficult to make. CMS's Physician Group Practice Demonstration is an example of the generated-savings model. It provides a framework for how such a model can be used for subsets of providers (see Box 3-2). Rather than comparing actual spending with a projection, the demonstration compares actual spending on the beneficiaries served by participating providers with that on beneficiaries who receive care from similar providers not participating in the demonstration. However, this method of overcoming the difficulties involved in developing accurate projections would not be available if all providers were included in the program.

Adequacy

Whether the generated-savings model can produce adequate resources for a reward pool is largely unknown. A conundrum could develop: rewards of a certain size might be required to motivate the implementation of meaningful efficiency initiatives, but until significant efficiencies had been realized, the reward pool might be inadequate to support significant bonuses.

BOX 3-2   The Physician Group Practice Demonstration: Example of a Generated-Savings Reward Pool

The Physician Group Practice Demonstration is Medicare's first pay-for-performance program for physicians. The program was mandated by the Medicare, Medicaid, and State Children's Health Insurance Program Benefits Improvement and Protection Act of 2000 and became operational in April 2005. Under this project, ten large group practices (consisting of at least 200 physicians each) are encouraged to improve both clinical quality and efficiency in health care services for Medicare fee-for-service beneficiaries. The 3-year program is aimed at improving coordination of Part A and Part B services, investing in structural and process efficiencies, and rewarding improved outcomes (CMS, 2005). Physicians will continue to be paid on a fee-for-service basis; they may earn additional rewards based on their results, but only if they achieve savings as compared with a projected annual target. By law, the demonstration is budget neutral. Accordingly, the performance rewards are derived from the savings.

SOURCE: CMS, 2005.

Stability

This model could prove fairly unstable in that the difference between projected and actual spending could vary significantly from year to year. It is difficult to predict year-to-year spending increases with any degree of accuracy because so many factors affect spending, often in ways that are not fully understood.

Fairness

Providers would probably consider this approach more equitable than the existing-funds model. They would reap the benefits of their actions directly, in that the savings generated by their efforts to improve would be distributed back to them. However, the generation of savings might depend critically on the cooperation of multiple providers across settings within a community, which might be difficult to achieve. Initially at least, this could be problematic if the savings generated by all provider settings were consolidated into one reward pool, and adequate performance measures that could be used to allocate rewards were lacking for some types of providers. Accrued savings could be attributed and awarded to individual providers, but this would be an extremely complex undertaking fraught with difficulties, including those associated with the calculation of savings and attribution of care to a single provider. Under this model, multiple smaller reward pools might be considered fairer for properly attributing savings.

Variations across regions in levels of spending and the pace of spending growth also relate to perceptions of fairness. Providers in regions with relatively low spending levels might argue that they had already achieved a desirable level of efficiency and had little scope for reducing their rate of spending growth. If the reward pool were generated largely from high-spending regions but the bonuses were concentrated in more efficient regions, many of which deliver relatively high-quality care (Fisher et al., 2003), provider dissatisfaction could emerge in the former areas.

Impact

The generated-savings model places great emphasis on efficiencies and program savings. This emphasis could have a negative impact on clinical quality. It is therefore important that the bonus or reward system under such a model emphasize clinical quality and patient-centeredness. This could be accomplished through the reward distribution design by establishing thresholds for these two domains that would have to be exceeded before a provider received a reward for either the level of or improvement in efficiency (see Chapter 4). To the extent that efficiencies can best be achieved by providers working together, this approach could indirectly encourage providers to collaborate to generate these savings and individual physicians to form larger group practices through formal or informal affiliations. This approach would also allow communities to self-organize at the market level to work toward a common objective. While this approach may appear plausible in any care setting, however, in reality such a model has been implemented only at the hospital level (see Box 3-3). Sparse empirical evidence exists to support the transfer of this approach to a larger-scale effort.

Direct Investment

The options discussed thus far are initially budget neutral, involving no new money up front. The direct-investment model differs in this regard.

The Institute of Medicine's (IOM's) *Crossing the Quality Chasm* report recommended that a discrete number of common, high-burden chronic conditions serve as leverage points for achieving rapid and widespread improvements in the six quality aims of health care (IOM, 2001). A subsequent IOM report, *Priority Areas for National Action: Transforming Health Care Quality*, recommended 20 priority conditions or areas in which to proceed (IOM, 2003). Continuing with this path, the committee considered whether initial pay-for-performance strategies should be directed at these priority

---

BOX 3-3   Excellus Blue Cross Blue Shield: Combination of Generated Savings and Withholds for Reward Pools

In an example of funding based partially on cost savings, Excellus Blue Cross Blue Shield of Rochester, New York, partnered with 900 physicians of the Rochester Individual Practice Association to reward providers who met standards of clinical quality, cost savings, and patient experience of care. Excellus looked at the years 2001 and 2002 as a base. It then invested $1.1 million into the program each year, with a positive return on investment of 2–3 dollars for every dollar invested. The program also created a bonus pool of up to $15 million based on a combination of withholds and shared savings. Thus this program shows elements of all three short-term models discussed in this chapter, although in this example, it is used specifically to illustrate how cost savings can be employed in the funding of a reward pool. With this combination of withholds and shared savings, 8 percent of physicians' reimbursement was at risk, but they could receive a return of 50–150 percent depending on their performance.

SOURCE: AIS, 2004.

---

areas. The assumption behind doing so would be that investments in upstream preventive services, such as cancer screenings, and high quality for individuals in the initial stages of a chronic condition could generate significant downstream savings that could fund future pay-for-performance initiatives for other health conditions. The goal would be to target high-value interventions and to reward providers for delivering evidence-based services.

Adequacy

An investment of any size in a pay-for-performance reward pool would constitute adding new money to the health finance system. The size of the investment, however, could vary and would have to be sufficient to stimulate the desired level of activity. Providers could be given funds up front to work on specific conditions, such as the priority areas noted above, with the payments not being linked to performance, so as to initiate the program and encourage providers to focus on these areas. Subsequent payments could be tied to the achievement of specific treatment goals for that limited number of conditions. (See Box 3-4 for an example of direct investment for specific clinical conditions.)

BOX 3-4 HealthPartners: Use of Comprehensive Quality Standards in Direct-Investment Models

HealthPartners is a consortium of nonprofit, consumer-run health care organizations in Minnesota, including a health plan that covers nearly one-fourth of the residents of the Minneapolis–St. Paul metropolitan area. In 1997, HealthPartners began rewarding primary care physicians for achieving specific clinical quality performance goals through its Outcomes Recognition Program. In contrast to some programs, HealthPartners did not attempt to create a budget-neutral approach— any provider achieving goals on health outcomes received awards. Most of the outcome goals depended on an "all-or-none" approach. That is, for a physician to receive a reward for one condition, the individual patient had to meet standards for multiple outcomes. For example, "Optimal Diabetes Care" required that at least 30 percent of a group's HealthPartners adult (aged 18–75) patients with diabetes have all cardiovascular risk factors optimally managed. To meet this comprehensive standard, patients had to have blood sugar (HbA_1c) levels less than or equal to 8 percent, LDL cholesterol less than 130 mg/dl, and blood pressure under 130/85 mmHg. Moreover, patients had to be nonsmokers, and those older than age 40 had to be taking aspirin daily. In 2004, 3 of the 26 eligible primary group practices were able to achieve this standard for diabetes care.

SOURCE: Apland and Amundson, 2005.

Stability

In and of itself, the pool under a direct-investment model is initially stable in that it represents a set amount of funds calibrated to meet the needs of the program. The pool size could expand if savings were reinvested into the program, much as in the generated-savings model. Caution is in order, however, because the current evidence base provides few examples of large positive returns on investments of this sort. There has been some experience with this general model in the private sector that offers insight into the process of implementation, operation, and lessons learned. However, a significant challenge remains because this strategy requires new money from the outset, which would be difficult to obtain in the current fiscal climate. Realistically, if this model were to be financially sustainable in the long run, it would require that both clinical effectiveness (i.e., meeting clinical quality targets) and efficiency be achieved.

Fairness

This option is characterized by a high degree of fairness because while not all providers would be eligible for initial rewards, the funds used to support the program would not come from any one provider group.

Impact

The impact of this model is unclear. If successful, it would directly affect the clinical quality of care delivered to beneficiaries for the targeted priority conditions because specific care processes for these conditions would attract more attention. Use of this model is supported by the fact that Medicare payments are highly concentrated on a few conditions. For example, 70 percent of Medicare inpatient spending is made for beneficiaries who have, either singly or in combination, three chronic conditions—chronic heart failure, coronary artery disease, and diabetes (MedPAC, 2005) (see the discussion of rewarding by condition in Chapter 4). By focusing on a few high-cost conditions, providers could have a significant impact on both savings and clinical quality.

However, one serious concern with this approach is the possibility that certain providers might choose to avoid patients with these conditions so they would not be compelled to participate in a pay-for-performance program. Of course, if the rewards were substantial, providers might be attracted to the program, thereby improving access for those with these chronic conditions. A direct-investment model in which savings went into a common reward pool that was allocated only in cases in which the patient received all necessary care from all providers could promote shared accountability for and coordination of patient care since each provider's bonus would be tied to the performance of all. However, there are few established models for distributing rewards in this manner across multiple providers. Reward pools might be diluted if the money were allocated across a large number of providers. (Distribution issues are discussed in greater detail in Chapter 4.)

Evaluation of Short-Term Alternatives

As described above, the committee examined a number of alternatives for funding an initial pay-for-performance program in Medicare, weighing the strengths and weaknesses of each. A good deal of uncertainty surrounds all of these alternatives. Moreover, the committee recognizes that these models have often been used in combination, and that new strategies may emerge as experience enriches the knowledge base. The committee evaluated each with respect to the four overarching criteria it deemed important to the choice of a funding source: adequacy, stability, fairness, and impact. A summary of the alternatives and their characteristics according to these four criteria appears in Table 3-3.

In light of this comparison, the committee makes the following recommendation:

> **Recommendation 2: Congress should derive initial funding (over the next 3–5 years) for a pay-for-performance program in Medicare largely from existing funds.**

- Congress should create provider-specific pools from a reduction in the base Medicare payments for each class of providers (hospitals, skilled nursing facilities, Medicare Advantage plans, dialysis facilities, home health agencies, and physicians).
- Congress should ensure that these pools are large enough to create adequate motivation for improved performance on selected measures. Because of unique challenges of physician payment relating to the sustainable growth rate (SGR), investment dollars may be necessary to create adequate resources to effect change.
- Initial funding should be budget conscious in taking into account the resources needed for both funding the pools and implementing the program.

The committee recognizes that generation of a reward pool with existing funds is useful for an initial pay-for-performance program, but should be only be a short-term solution while alternative funding sources are explored. The feasibility of other funding approaches and the savings realized from efficiency improvement should be evaluated over the next 3–5 years.

The committee concluded that the generated-savings model on its own is currently limited by difficulties with prediction and is not sustainable, but has great potential. As a result, the committee proposes that efforts to test and demonstrate ways of making this source of funds work be mounted and aggressively pursued. Based upon the findings from those efforts, funds generated by increased efficiency should be used as a supplemental source in the creation of subsequent funding pools. The committee also concluded that the direct-investment model is inadequate on its own because of difficulties in finding sufficient new money for initial investment, as well as related concerns regarding the attribution of care. However, the committee did recognize that some new funds may be needed in addition to existing sources to initiate the program up front.

TABLE 3-3 Comparison of Initial Funding Options

Criterion	Existing Funds	Generated Savings	Direct Investment
Adequacy	**Mixed**—Updates and base payment reductions are too small to motivate some providers and will need time to accumulate to viable size. Will be adequate if pool is created to a level that is predetermined.	**Low**—Amount required to motivate change is unknown, and amount of savings is largely unpredictable. Also, no start-up funds present to initiate changes.	**Low**—Places new money into the system, but finding a source of new money in the current fiscal climate that will be adequate to motivate all providers is highly unlikely.
Stability	**Moderate**—Low complexity and possibility of immediate implementation, but high variability in size of update. Confounded in light of negative updates.	**Low**—Difficult to predict spending increases, requires complex formulas to calculate savings, and can fluctuate greatly from year to year.	**Low**—Pool initially stable since has known source and size, but return on investment is unknown, and sustainability is uncertain.
Fairness	**Moderate**—Some providers are precluded from program, and not all get updates (or equivalent updates).	**Moderate**—Some providers are precluded, but others may directly reap the benefit of their efficiencies. Complicated by sharing of pool, attribution, and comparison groups.	**High**—Fair in that source does not affect those who cannot participate.
Impact	Reduces already low payment rates. May create access problems.	Greater incentive for savings and efficiency. May encourage care coordination.	Specific conditions are targeted for attention. Potential exists for adverse selection. May promote care coordination.

In considering geographic levels for funding pools, the committee concluded that initial reward pools should be established by provider setting at the national level because of concerns about complexity and attribution at the regional level, as well as the fairness of creating an aggregate pool for all provider settings. While the committee acknowledges that pools created at the provider setting level would do little to foster increased care coordination, it also recognizes that the current payment system does even less in this regard. Furthermore, the creation of a single aggregate pool would likely not be acceptable to major stakeholders because of perceptions of unfairness, the inability to attribute care accurately, and the need for the development of more sophisticated measures that would specifically address care coordination.

The existing-funds model is consistent with the goal of linking larger proportions of payment to performance. Again, while recommended as an initial approach to funding, the committee recognizes that this model represents a short-term solution and that other strategies will have to be tested and considered as new challenges arise in Medicare pay-for-performance programs.

LONG-TERM FUNDING

The prior discussion of alternative models for funding pay-for-performance programs constitutes a plan for incremental reforms. The committee has presented these alternatives and made its final recommendation while fully acknowledging the strengths and weaknesses of each model. The committee also recognizes that each of these alternatives may be a transitional step while long-term funding options are explored. In essence, these short-term strategies should be viewed as initial building blocks that could help move Medicare toward future funding alternatives and payment policies that would represent more robust approaches for aligning payment incentives with higher-quality care.

In considering the scope of the reward pools, the committee has recommended separate pools for each major provider setting. In the long term, however, the committee believes that as measurement becomes more sophisticated and it becomes possible to evaluate performance for episodes of care and for all care given to those with significant chronic conditions, it will make sense to consolidate the multiple reward pools into a single national pool. However, the committee recognizes the need to reconcile this approach with the fact that provider payments in Medicare (such as from Part A and Part B) are currently unlinked.

Recommendation 3: Congress should give the Secretary of DHHS the authority to aggregate the pools for different care settings into one consolidated pool from which all providers would be rewarded when the development of new performance measures allows for shared accountability and more coordinated care across provider settings.

CONCLUSION

Pay for performance represents a major shift from the status quo, one that is likely to be met with marked resistance. The committee has recommended that the initial pool for pay for performance come from a reduction in base Medicare payments, with the current update mechanism being retained. CMS should also experiment with the generated-savings model as soon as possible. In certain areas, investments of new funds may be unavoidable. The committee has also recommended the initial creation of multiple reward pools by care setting that, in the long term, would be aggregated into one large pool from which all providers could earn rewards.

The issues examined in this chapter related to the funding of a pay-for-performance program in Medicare set the stage for discussion of many of the policy implications of subsequent decisions about the implementation of such a program. While some of these considerations have been touched upon in this chapter, separate discussion of the distribution of these funds is presented next in Chapter 4, and overarching concerns regarding the implementation of the program are addressed in Chapter 5.

REFERENCES

AAFP (American Academy of Family Physicians). 2005 (July 1). *Position Statement from the American Academy of Family Physicians: Per Family Physicians: Medicare Value Purchasing Act Misses the Mark.* Unpublished.

ACHP (Alliance of Community Health Plans). 2004. *Position Statement of the Alliance of Community Health Plans: Four Principles for "Payment-for-Performance" in Medicare.* [Online]. Available: http://www.achp.org/news/article.asp?nyear=2004&article_id=97 [accessed June 12, 2006].

ACHP. 2005 (June 28). *Position Statement of the Alliance of Community Health Plans.* Unpublished.

ACOG (American College of Obstetricians and Gynecologists). 2005. *Position Statement of the American College of Obstetricians and Gynecologists: Pay for Performance (P4P).* Unpublished.

ACP (American College of Physicians). 2005 (March 15). *Position Statement of the American College of Physicians for the Record of the Hearing on Measuring Quality and Efficiency of Care in Medicare.* Unpublished.

AIS (Atlantic Information Services, Inc.). 2004. *Case Studies in Health Plan Pay-for-Performance Programs*. Washington, DC: AIS.

AMA (American Medical Association). 2005. *Position Statement from the American Medical Association: Pay-for-Performance Principles and Guidelines*. [Online]. Available: http://www.ama-assn.org/meetings/public/annual 05/bot5a05fin.doc [accessed June 12, 2006].

Apland BA, Amundson GM. 2005. Financial incentives: An indispensable element for quality improvement. *Patient Safety and Quality Healthcare* 2(5):6–8.

Bailit Health Purchasing LLC. 2002. *Provider Incentive Models for Improving Quality of Care*. Washington, DC: Academy for Health Services Research and Health Policy.

Baker G, Carter B. 2005. *Provider Pay-for-Performance Incentive Programs: 2004 National Study Results*. San Francisco, CA: Med-Vantage, Inc.

CMS (Centers for Medicare and Medicaid Services). 2005. *CMS Fact Sheet*. [Online]. Available: http://www.premierinc.com/advocacy/issues/medicare/05/physician-group-practice-fact-sheet-0105.pdf#search='Physician%20Group%20Practice%20Demonstration' [accessed March 2, 2006].

de Brantes F, Galvin RS, Lee TH. 2003. Bridges to excellence: Building a business case for quality care. *Journal of Clinical Outcomes Management* 10(8):439–446.

Fisher ES, Wennberg DE, Stukel TA, Gottlieb DJ, Lucas FL, Pinder EL. 2003. The implications of regional variations in Medicare spending. Part 1: The content, quality, and accessibility of care. *Annals of Internal Medicine* 138(4):273–287.

IOM (Institute of Medicine). 2001. *Crossing the Quality Chasm: A New Health System for the 21st Century*. Washington, DC: National Academy Press.

IOM. 2003. *Priority Areas for National Action: Transforming Health Care Quality*. Adams K, Corrigan JM, eds. Washington, DC: The National Academies Press.

MedPAC (Medicare Payment Advisory Commission). 2005. *MedPAC Data Runs*. Washington, DC: MedPAC.

MedPAC. 2006. *Report to the Congress: Medicare Payment Policy*. Washington, DC: MedPAC.

Nussbaum S. 2005. *Testimony to Medicare Payment Advisory Commission*. [Online]. Available: http://www.medpac.gov/public_meetings/transcripts/0905_allcombined_transc.pdf [accessed August 2, 2006].

Roland M. 2004. Linking physicians' pay to the quality of care: A major experiment in the United Kingdom. *New England Journal of Medicine* 351(14):1448–1454.

Rosenthal MB, Fernandopulle R, Song HR, Landon B. 2004. Paying for quality: Providers' incentives for quality improvement. *Health Affairs* 23(2):127–141.

Smith PC, York N. 2004. Quality incentives: The case of U.K. general practitioners—An ambitious U.K. quality improvement initiative offers the potential for enormous gains in the quality of primary health care. *Health Affairs* 23(3):112–118.

4

Distribution of Rewards

CHAPTER SUMMARY

The preceding chapter discussed the advantages and disadvantages of several approaches to funding pay for performance within the Medicare program and offered rationales for both short- and long-term strategies. This chapter focuses on how rewards could be distributed to providers. Also discussed are general guidelines for designing an incentive-based system, such as what aspects of care to reward, what measures to reward, and how large payments must be to have the desired effect. Issues dealing with the implementation of such a system are assessed in Chapter 5.

As summarized in Chapter 2, the current fee-for-service payment system has both strengths and weaknesses. Among its weaknesses is that it provides incentives for overuse of services and fails to impose systematic penalties for misuse or underuse of medical care. Embedded in the system, moreover, are incentives to use certain procedures over other, less costly ones that may be equally or more effective. Together these weaknesses create an environment in which the provision of higher-quality care at lower cost is not the standard.

The health care delivery system has evolved over time with better understanding of diseases and the human body and the development of new technologies and procedures. Provision of medical care is significantly different from what it was 40 years ago when Medicare began; yet the fee-for-service payment system has changed little, except for the replacement of cost-based prospective payments. Attempts to modify the payment system—such as efforts to encourage coordinated or managed care—have been met with limited success. Pay for performance is a critical tool that can, if implemented carefully, begin to address the undesirable consequences of the fee-for-service system.

This chapter addresses options for distributing rewards to high-performing providers. First it addresses the question of just what should be rewarded under a pay-for-performance program. Next it examines various design elements, such as how to measure performance and what basis to use for the distribution of rewards. The chapter then looks at how to operationalize these design elements, describing various models for assigning and distributing rewards to providers. There are many nuances involved in the design of any pay-for-performance program. The discussion in this chapter is intended to illustrate the challenges designers will face.

WHAT TO REWARD

Identifying Domains of Care

Pay for performance should provide incentives for delivering higher-quality care to achieve all six aims for health care identified in the Institute of Medicine's (IOM's) *Quality Chasm* report: safety, effectiveness, patient-centeredness, timeliness, efficiency, and equity (IOM, 2001). Many physicians and health care organizations are skeptical that reliable and valid performance measures can be developed for complex clinical processes. They are equally doubtful that payment incentives can be put in place that will reward performance in ways that affect what truly matters: improving the health of patients. Another major challenge facing designers of pay-for-performance programs is guarding against the possibility that efforts to improve one domain of care may adversely affect other domains. For example, many purchasers are concerned that performance measures emphasizing enhanced clinical quality will lead to an unrestrained growth in costs and a minimal effort to reduce current waste and inefficiencies.

Any pay-for-performance program must address these concerns by clarifying the goals and objectives of new payment mechanisms. In considering how to do so, the committee drew on the vision set forth in the *Quality Chasm* report, in particular the six aims cited above. Current performance measurement approaches are focused heavily on clinical effectiveness. While this domain is crucial to improving the overall quality of health care, an overemphasis on clinical effectiveness risks defining good care too narrowly by failing to consider the perspectives of patients, their families, and society as a whole, as well as limitations in resource availability. Pay for performance should be based on performance measures that are aligned with long-term goals for improving all aspects of quality that foster improved patient outcomes within an environment of limited resources. In its consideration of initial measures that would ensure high quality and improve the value of health care investments, the committee found it convenient to consolidate the six aims of the *Quality Chasm* report into three broader domains that should serve as the foundation for new payment incentives: clinical quality, patient-centered care, and efficiency.

Recommendation 4: In designing a pay-for-performance program, the Secretary of DHHS should initially reward health care that is of high clinical quality, patient-centered, and efficient.

The committee believes efforts to improve quality should focus initially on these three broad domains, eventually disaggregating the focus to ensure that all six quality aims are adequately addressed. This consolidation into three domains should not be viewed as diminishing the value of the six aims. Rather, this initial approach is intended to streamline the complex task of implementing pay for performance while at the same time ensuring that performance is considered comprehensively.

Domain-Based Rewards

There are numerous ways a reward pool could be divided among the three domains of clinical quality, patient-centeredness, and efficiency. The following discussion illustrates simplified versions of the options the committee considered.

Option 1: Even Distribution

The total dollars in the reward pool could be split evenly across the domains. For instance, if $3 billion were available to distribute, $1 billion could be allocated for achievements in each domain.

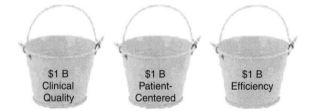

Even distribution would signal that policy makers regarded improved performance in all three domains to be equally important. However, this option may not be advisable if robust and sufficient measures are unavailable for all domains.

Option 2: Uneven Distribution

A second option would be to distribute the rewards unevenly, emphasizing some domains over others. For example, $1.5 billion could be designated to reward clinical quality, $1 billion patient-centeredness, and $0.5 billion efficiency.

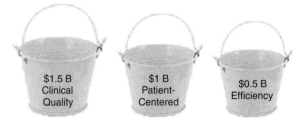

This approach would be appropriate if policy makers deemed improvement in certain domains more important than that in others. This option might also be advisable if the validity and comprehensiveness of measures across domains differed or if larger incentives were found to be necessary to motivate equal improvement in all three domains.

Conclusion

Little objective evidence exists to inform a judgment about the appropriate distribution of rewards across the three domains. Nor is there a clear consensus on the relative priorities for improvement in each domain to guide the allocation decision. Practical considerations—namely, that there are few well-developed measures available for patient-centeredness and efficiency (see the discussion below)—led the committee to conclude that, initially at least, most of the reward pool should be allocated to incentives for improved clinical quality, where applicable. Improvements in each domain would ideally be made with consideration of the others, with the goal of improving all three. The Secretary of the Department of Health and Human Services (DHHS) should decide exactly how much is to be allocated to each domain. The distribution of payment across the domains should be adjusted as the program develops. As measures and pubic reporting initiatives supporting a pay-for-performance program evolve, policies, and therefore reimbursement levels, will also need to be adjusted.

Improvement and Excellence

Pay-for-performance programs have generally been structured to reward one or both of two possible dimensions: improvement and excellence.

Improvement

Under a system that rewarded improvement, providers would be eligible for a reward if their performance improved significantly. Improvement is measured in many ways; one approach that is employed currently by the Centers for Medicare and Medicaid Services (CMS) is the percentage reduction in the failure rate, defined as the difference between perfect and actual performance.[1] Under this method, even very high-performing providers would have the ability to earn rewards because the higher a provider's initial performance was, the smaller the absolute increase in performance would have to be to achieve any particular decrease in the failure rate. For example, if the baseline performance measure for hospital A were 80 percent, its failure rate would be 20 percent. If 1 year later hospital A's performance had improved by 4 percent to 84 percent, the reduction in its failure rate would be 20 percent. Hospital B, with an initial performance score of 40 percent (and a failure rate of 60 percent) would have to improve its performance by 12 percent to 52 percent to achieve a 20 percent reduction in its failure rate. However, the reduction in failure rate is not a perfect measure. It might take more resources and be more difficult for hospital A to improve performance than for hospital B. And even if possible, 100 percent may not be desirable.

Excellence

A system designed to reward excellence would reward only those providers who attained or exceeded a specified threshold of performance. In other words, only those that truly were among the best performers would be rewarded for delivering high-quality care. The threshold could be an aggregate or average of several measures. There could also be several thresholds, all or some of which would have to be met to receive any award.

Analysis and Conclusion

Providing rewards for improvement has the advantage of offering incentives to all providers to improve their performance. A criticism of an approach that rewards only improvement, however, is that some providers with truly excellent performance would receive no rewards, while others who even after significant improvement were performing at a mediocre level would benefit. This situation might persist only for a few years if the required levels of improvement were significant (e.g., an annual 15 percent reduction in the failure rate) because after several years of such sizable improvements, initially poor performers would by default become high performers. Another concern with rewarding only improvement is gaming. For example, it would be necessary to guard against a situation in which a mediocre performer earned a reward for improving significantly in year 1,

---

[1]Reduction in failure rate is the change in performance from baseline to follow-up, divided by the difference between baseline and perfect (100 percent) performance.

then let performance slide in year 2, and again obtained a reward in year 3 for significant improvement (much of which had been rewarded in the first year). To prevent this, the reduction in the failure rate could be measured from the provider's previous highest level of performance.

If the system rewarded only excellence, providers that were well below the threshold for excellence might conclude that, because they had little chance of reaching the threshold, investments to improve specific areas of quality would not be worth the effort or cost. Another concern with rewarding only excellence is that rewards, at least initially, might be concentrated geographically, which could undercut support for a pay-for-performance initiative. On the other hand, a strength of a system that rewarded excellence would be that it would send a clear signal as to what the nation expects from a high-performing health care system.

Recognizing the advantages and limitations of each approach, the committee concluded that a combined approach should be taken:

Recommendation 5: The Secretary of DHHS should design a pay-for-performance program that initially rewards both providers who improve performance significantly and those who achieve high performance.

Under such a combined approach, providers at all levels would be most likely to find at least one of the two goals within reach. The committee expects that the distribution of the aggregate reward pool between encouraging improvement and rewarding excellence will shift over time. As providers make significant improvements in their performance, the fraction of the pool devoted to rewarding excellence should grow. This shift may occur rather slowly because as the vast majority of providers reach and sustain good performance according to certain measures, new measures focusing on different aspects of quality should be introduced into the system. This shift should be monitored and distribution adjusted in evaluations of any pay-for-performance program (see Chapter 6).

WHAT MEASURES SHOULD BE USED FOR REWARD-BASED PAYMENTS

Identifying Measure Sets for Assessing Performance

How payments are distributed within each of the three domains depends in part on the measures employed. Certain disease conditions or care settings may be preferable starting points because of the availability of reliable measures and the expectation that significant improvements in performance can be achieved.

If rewards are to be based on provider performance, the system must be capable of reliably defining and transparently identifying good care. However, the IOM report *Performance Measurement: Accelerating Improvement* (IOM, 2006) identified gaps in currently available measures. First, measures for some of the six quality aims set forth in the *Quality Chasm* report (IOM, 2001) are lacking; current measures focus largely on effectiveness. Second, currently available measures do not adequately reflect health care across the life span; for example, few measures adequately characterize care at the end of life, as compared with the many measures for living with chronic disease. A third limitation is that measures—which are usually categorized into indicators of structure, process, or outcomes—are heavily process-based (Bradley et al., 2006). Structural measures evaluate the physical structures associated with care delivery, process measures assess how care is actually delivered, and outcome measures consider the health of a patient as a result of care received. To better characterize health care delivery, more measures that can capture relationships among structure, process, and outcomes need to be developed (IOM, 2006). Because only a small portion of care delivery is currently being measured, pay for performance necessarily will be limited initially to rewarding specific subsets of care.

Available measures for each of the three domains are far from being adequate to support a comprehensive pay-for-performance program. Clinical quality measures are currently further along than those for patient-centeredness, while efficiency measures are still largely under development. Existing measure sets are organized largely by care setting. Building on the starter set of measures presented in the *Performance Measurement* report, the committee believes the measures presented in Table 4-1 should be used in the short term for a pay-for-performance program with the exception of the Minimum Data Set, which should not be used in pay for performance to provide incentives for skilled nursing facilities (see Chapter 5). As discussed in the *Performance Measurement* report, the following criteria were considered in choosing the starter set:

- Scientific soundness
- Feasibility
- Importance
- Alignment
- Comprehensiveness

Given that current measures were developed by care setting, rewards will initially have to be distributed by setting until more measures across sites of care and across time are developed. These measures were current as of August 2005 and should be considered the minimum for reporting. Upon

TABLE 4-1 Recommended Starter Set of Performance Measures

Ambulatory Care	**Ambulatory care Quality Alliance (26)** Prevention measures[a] (7), coronary artery disease[a] (3), heart failure[a] (2), diabetes[a] (6), asthma[a] (2), depression[a] (2), prenatal care[a] (2), quality measures addressing overuse or misuse (2) **Ambulatory Care Survey** CAHPS[b] Clinician and Group Survey: getting care quickly, getting needed care, how well providers communicate, health promotion and education, shared decision making, knowledge of medical history, how well office staff communicate
Acute Care	**Hospital Quality Alliance (22)** Acute coronary syndrome[a] (7), heart failure[a] (3), pneumonia[a] (6), smoking cessation[a] (3), surgical infection prevention[a] (from the Surgical Care Improvement Project) (3) **Structural measures** (computerized provider order entry, intensive care unit intensivists, evidence-based hospital referrals) **Hospital CAHPS** Patient communication with physicians, patient communication with nurses, responsiveness of hospital staff, cleanliness/noise level of physical environment, pain control, communications about medicines, discharge information
Health Plans and Accountable Health Organizations	**Health Plan Employer Data and Information Set (HEDIS) (61)** Integrated delivery systems (health maintenance organizations): effectiveness (26), access/availability of care (8), satisfaction with the experience of care (4), health plan stability (2), use of service (15), cost of care, informed health care choices, health plan descriptive information (6) Preferred provider organizations within Medicare Advantage: selected administrative data and hybrid measures **Ambulatory Care Survey** CAHPS Health Plan Survey: getting care quickly, getting needed care, how well providers communicate, health plan paperwork, health plan customer service
Long-Term Care	**Minimum Data Set (15)** Long-term care (12), short-stay care (3) **Outcome and Assessment Information Set (11)** Ambulation/locomotion (1), transferring (1), toileting (1), pain (1), bathing (2), management of oral medications (1), acute care hospitalization (1), emergent care (1), confusion (1)
End-Stage Renal Disease	**National Healthcare Quality Report (5)** Transplant registry and results (2), dialysis effectiveness (2), mortality (1)
Longitudinal measures of outcomes and efficiency	1-year mortality, resource use, and functional status (SF-12) after acute myocardial infarction

[a]The committee recommends the aggregation of individual measures to patient-level composites for these areas.
[b]CAHPS = Consumer Assessment of Healthcare Providers and Systems.
SOURCE: IOM, 2006.

implementation of a pay-for-performance program, these measures should be updated to reflect the most up-to-date research.

Data Limitations

Data are collected using a variety of methods, primary among these being administrative claims and medical chart review. Retrievable electronic data are most frequently collected as administrative claims (commonly referred to as claims data or admin data), which are electronic medical bills submitted by providers to payers. Data derived from these electronic data include demographic information (e.g., patient age and gender), type of insurance coverage, and information regarding services received (e.g., cost, type, and place of service; lengths of stay; procedures performed; laboratory results; medications prescribed). In other cases, providers must abstract clinical data from individual medical charts (referred to as chart data) that currently are not retrievable electronically. Chart data include information such as results of diagnostic tests and procedures, medications, and therapeutic procedures.

There are many trade-offs involved in collecting data from the different sources, such as that between the burden of data collection and the value of the data collected. Collection of admin data requires only sorting of electronic data; thus this method is relatively quick and inexpensive. By contrast, collection of chart data requires that a nurse, physician, or some other certified person with medical knowledge go through each medical chart to abstract the data. This is not only time-consuming, but also costly. With regard to the importance of the data collected, admin data frequently do not adequately capture specific clinical information (e.g., whether cholesterol levels were controlled to less than 100 mg/dL) in the absence of electronic laboratory data. The latter can be found in some health plans and medical groups, but must otherwise be obtained through chart review. Judgments about the relative merits of admin versus chart data also need to take into account the frequency of collection and the accuracy and reliability of the data. Both modes of data collection are used; however, both are limited in the amount of information yielded, as well as the resources required to collect the data.

As pay-for-performance rewards can be based only on data that are collected, the data collection must be timely and capture the intermediate and ultimate outcomes of care while not imposing an undue burden on providers. Data systems are increasingly being designed with the capacity to collect more "meaningful" data electronically; this capability will be greatly accelerated by the adoption of health information technologies (see Chapter 5). The committee carefully weighed these considerations when assessing the types of measures on which to base pay for performance, but believes that obtaining meaningful data should not be precluded by the burden of data collection. This issue should be reevaluated as pay for performance and the measures on which it is based develop.

Rewarding by Condition

As noted in Chapter 3, the committee found that Medicare payments are focused on patients with specific common chronic conditions: 70 percent of Medicare inpatient spending is associated with the 32 percent of Medicare patients who have chronic heart failure, coronary artery disease, diabetes, or a combination of these conditions (MedPAC, 2005).[2] This finding suggests that initially, with respect to physician services, concentrating pay for performance on conditions (especially these three) would be practical.

There are two further reasons for pursuing a condition-based reward system. First, the measures in the starter set are often organized by condition and specific setting. Second, a provider-based system, the primary alternative, would not be practical because research has shown that providers who are high performers on one condition do not necessarily perform well on others (Jha et al., 2005). For example, a hospital can rank among the best for cardiac care and still provide suboptimal care for pneumonia patients.

It is important to note that the reward pools for various conditions would likely differ because, for example, improvements in one condition may be more difficult to achieve than those in others, the value of improvements may be greater for some conditions than for others, and the differences among providers may be less extreme for some conditions.

Rewarding Composite Measures of Care for Conditions

The committee believes measures should be bundled into composites for a given condition for each provider. The *Performance Measurement* report (IOM, 2006) proposed that measures for specific conditions be combined into a single composite per patient that would reflect whether the patient had received the minimum level of critical care required to treat a condition. For example, the individual measures of HbA$_1$c management, HbA$_1$c control, blood pressure management, lipid measurement, LDL cholesterol level, and eye exam would be grouped into a single composite for diabetes. To receive any aggregate reward, providers would have to exceed threshold levels for each measure. The *Performance Measurement* report also proposed that research be carried out to determine how each measure

---

[2]Data were derived from the Medicare 5 percent sample. Payment figures represent total physician fee schedule payments in the groups of diabetes, chronic heart failure, and coronary artery disease.

within a composite should be weighted. Measures of performance are often collected and reported by aggregating all the patients a provider treats, not by determining the total amount of care each individual patient received, because data are not currently adequate to characterize performance at the latter level (IOM, 2006).

Rewarding by Structure

Another option is to distribute rewards on the basis of structural measures of care. This approach might involve rewarding providers that have in place such structures as clinical care teams, care coordinators, and health information technology systems that are thought to improve the overall safety, timeliness, and efficiency of care. Some structural measures related to information technology, such as computerized provider order entry, intensive care unit intensivists, and evidence-based hospital referrals, are included in the starter set identified in the *Performance Measurement* report. Other structural measures, such as those for care coordination and nursing staff hours, are still largely under development (IOM, 2006). When ready, structural measures may provide incentives to create the infrastructure necessary to close current gaps in care. Rewarding by structure would be a promising way to foster more comprehensive systematic change in the health care delivery system.

HOW TO DISTRIBUTE REWARDS

Absolute Versus Relative Performance

Improvement and excellence can be rewarded on the basis of meeting predetermined, absolute levels of performance or performing well relative to other providers.

Absolute Thresholds

Absolute thresholds would establish minimum levels of performance providers would have to meet to be eligible for a reward. The use of absolute thresholds would allow providers to invest their resources with specific aims, as opposed to striving to achieve what would otherwise be an unknown moving target. A potential drawback of this approach is that if the provider community had an extremely high level of achievement, the reward pool would be distributed among a larger group of providers, reducing the amount of the individual rewards received. However, having a large proportion of providers meet thresholds would not be a negative outcome. If desired, a system could be designed to vary the size of the reward pool with the number of providers who performed well. In fact, this would be necessary if providers were to be certain of their reward for achieving the preset performance goals.

Tournament Style

Another option is a tournament-style or relative rewards structure, whereby rewards would be given to groups of providers who achieved a predetermined percentile ranking (e.g., 90th percentile), as opposed to a predetermined rank against measures as would be the case if absolute thresholds were used. Under this method, the best providers compared with their peers would be rewarded, and the situation in which everyone was above average—which can occur with absolute thresholds—could not arise. Because providers would be competing with each other and not attempting to achieve absolute thresholds, some lower performers might think that rewards were unattainable. On the other hand, this method could induce healthy competition among the best providers, potentially resulting in greater improvements than a system that failed to promote cutting-edge competition. Conversely, attempts to improve performance beyond a certain threshold (for example, from 98 percent to 100 percent) might produce diminishing returns and waste resources. Tournament-style rewards could also reward mediocre performance if the overall distribution of performance were low. For example, if the distribution of scores were low, providers in the 90th percentile might actually be delivering good care only 40 percent of the time, as defined by performance measures. The high level of uncertainty as to the amount of the rewards providers might receive could also be a disadvantage of this method because it might make providers hesitant to invest in quality improvement. In addition, a tournament-style reward system would limit the number of providers to whom rewards could be distributed. It could thus be viewed as disadvantageous to providers who believed improvements would be more difficult to make relative to other providers with whom they would be compared.

How High to Set Thresholds

There is little evidence that can be used for determining how high or low thresholds should be set in health care pay-for-performance programs to provide the most powerful incentive to improve. Given this lack of evidence, the committee proposes that CMS determine threshold levels. Clearly, thresholds should be set on the basis of clinical evidence and consensus as to what constitutes high-level performance and is reasonable to expect from providers. These levels of performance or percentiles for eligibility for rewards must be set in a timely fashion so providers can plan their quality improvement interventions in advance. Thresholds should also be constantly reviewed and set higher as long as average performance improves and higher levels of achievement are possible.

Graduated or Fixed Rewards

Distribution of rewards could be either graduated or fixed. In a graduated system, rewards would increase based on the amount of improvement or level of performance. With fixed rewards, the same amount would be distributed to all providers performing at or exceeding predetermined thresholds; below those thresholds, no rewards would be given. Either option could be used with both absolute and tournament-style thresholds, as well as with rewards based on both improvement and excellence. Absolute thresholds are used in the discussion here for simplicity; rewards based on both improvement and excellence are discussed for each option.

A graduated system for improvement could, for example, require a minimum 30 percent reduction in failure rate for a reward. To illustrate, Bloomfield Home for the Elderly (a hypothetical site) would receive $30 for improving from its baseline performance of 50 percent to 65 percent and $50 for improving to 85 percent, with scaled rewards in between that need not be linearly related to improvement (see Figure 4-1). If rewards were provided for excellence with a threshold of at least 65 percent, Bloomfield Home would receive $30 for its performance at 65 percent even if its baseline performance were 75 percent.

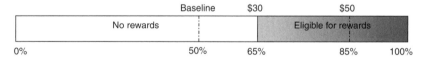

FIGURE 4-1   Eligibility for graduated rewards.

It is important to note that the maximum reward need not be provided for performance at 100 percent or a reduction in the failure rate of 100 percent. Under some measures, an increase from 90 to 100 percent might have only a marginal impact on health outcomes or might require investments not worth the benefits.

If rewards were fixed, Bloomfield Home would receive the same reward if its failure rate were reduced by 30 percent (from 50 to 65 percent) or by 90 percent (from 50 to 95 percent), as depicted in Figure 4-2. Below that fixed level, no rewards would be granted.

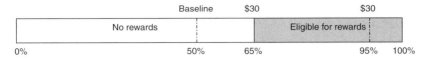

FIGURE 4-2   Eligibility for fixed rewards based on performance improvement.

If fixed rewards were provided for performance, Bloomfield Home would receive $50 whether its performance were 85 or 99 percent. It would receive nothing if its performance were 84.9 percent, as depicted in Figure 4-3.

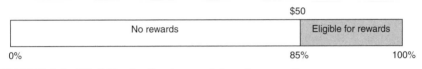

FIGURE 4-3   Eligibility for fixed rewards based on excellence.

A combination of fixed and graduated rewards might also be appropriate when linked to clinical conditions associated with the measure. For example, fixed rewards could be used for conditions for which there are continuous clinical benefits associated with additional gains (e.g., reduced postsurgical infection rates). On the other hand, graduated rewards could be used in cases where the additional clinical benefits diminish after a certain threshold is attained (e.g., HbA$_1$c management). In conclusion, the committee found that variable rewards would offer the advantage of motivating larger numbers of providers while giving the largest rewards to those whose performance was best and might be used more frequently than fixed rewards, if deemed appropriate.

Penalties for Lack of Improvement

To this point, rewards have been discussed on the basis of performing well (excellence) and upgrading performance within a given time period (improvement). What has not been discussed is what happens if a provider not only continues to perform poorly, but in fact allows performance to deteriorate. This issue must be considered in designing a pay-for-performance program.

One option is to penalize providers who exhibit the worst performance or the least effort to improve. The size of the penalties could be determined in a manner similar to that for rewards. The penalty amounts could be returned to the Medicare trust funds, CMS could distribute the penalty money to high-performing providers as additional rewards, or the penalty money could be held in an escrow account that poor-quality providers could earn back upon improved performance, among other options.

It is important to note that the committee recommends funding pay for performance initially out of base payments, so that all Medicare providers would contribute to the reward pool (see Chapter 3 for a discussion of the reward pool and Chapter 5 for a discussion of participation in pay for performance). Therefore, those who consistently performed poorly would pay penalties in addition to the reduction in their base payments.

A system with penalties would create stronger incentives for good, or at least adequate, performance and continued attention to improved performance. However, such a system could generate considerable resistance among providers. Providers who were not confident of their ability to improve might refuse to participate.

An alternative would be not to impose penalties on providers with very poor or deteriorating performance. The argument in favor of this approach is that providers would already be experiencing reductions in their base payments and that this should give them incentive enough to improve. Moreover, seriously deficient providers should probably be either removed from Medicare participation or be required to engage in a quality improvement program managed by their local Quality Improvement Organization.

Definition of Comparison Groups for the Purpose of Determining Rewards for Providers

Pay-for-performance rewards would be distributed within groups of providers. These groups can be defined according to a number of characteristics that are not mutually exclusive, such as procedure or service, setting of care, specialty, and location. Certain procedures and types of care are provided in a variety of settings. For example, minor surgery might be provided in outpatient hospital departments, ambulatory surgical centers, or physician offices; post–acute care might be provided by a skilled nursing facility unit in an acute care hospital, a free-standing skilled nursing facility, or a home health agency. The comparison group for pay for performance could be all those who provide a particular service or all those who provide the service in similar settings or have the same training. While comparisons across all care settings or specialties would appear to be the most equitable approach, comparable measures may not be available for all settings and specialties. Differentiation across settings, however, could prove to be problematic because providers might seek to define the comparison group very narrowly. For example, some might argue that comparisons should be only among hospitals of a certain size (e.g., over versus under 200 beds) or type (e.g., teaching versus nonteaching).

For a program such as Medicare, which operates throughout a nation in which market conditions, practice patterns, and other circumstances vary considerably from one locality to another, the geographic scope of a pay-for-performance program becomes an issue. Central is the question of whether comparisons should be made across the nation or regionally when rewarding excellence. If providers were compared nationally, the system would ensure that high-quality care was defined in a uniform way across the country. Furthermore, national standards preclude the inequity inherent in rewarding top performers in a region with low average performance while denying rewards to providers with better performance who happen to be located in regions with high overall performance. National comparisons might undercut support for a pay-for-performance program if few providers in certain regions received rewards. However, comparisons that focused only on a subset of the country might not adequately address disparities in performance arising from regional variations in practice patterns. If significant regional differences (such as those found in the Dartmouth Atlas project for acute myocardial infarction and chronic disease care) are found to exist in the performance being measured, CMS should consider a blend of regional and national comparison groups. Over time, however, a uniform national comparison should be used.

Models for Distribution

As discussed previously, rewards should be focused on the three domains of performance by setting of care and by condition. The next question for consideration is how the reward pools for improvement and excellence should be allocated among these domains. There are many feasible options for distribution, three of which are discussed below.

Option 1

For both improvement and excellence, each of the three domains could be given equal weight through a simple point system such as that shown below, which provides the maximum possible points possible for each category:

Models of Distribution

Clinical Quality	Patient-Centeredness	Efficiency
Excellence—16.67 points	Excellence—16.67 points	Excellence—16.67 points
Improvement—16.67 points	Improvement—16.67 points	Improvement—16.67 points

Under this example, a specific dollar amount or share of the reward pool would be attached to each point. Provider payments under this system would, therefore, be based on performing well in any of the three domains. Such a system would provide rewards to providers with inconsistent performance—for example, those delivering clinically high-quality care very inefficiently. Those who had the greatest improvement and highest level of excellence across all domains would receive the largest rewards.

Option 2

An alternative system might require that a minimum threshold level of excellence be reached in one, several, or all domains for a provider to receive any points in the other domains. For example, a provider might have to score at or above the 50th percentile on clinical quality to receive points for efficiency. This option could ensure that rewards for high-quality care would not be given to those with excessive resource use. Such a system would create a considerably smaller pool of eligible providers, especially if there were thresholds for each domain.

Option 3

The final option would be to allocate the points in option 1 unequally. This system would reflect practical considerations, such as the fact that measures are less available and robust in some domains than others and that in the early years, one might want to emphasize improvement more than excellence to motivate the most providers possible and counteract pushback from low-performing geographic regions. Over time, the allocation of points could be changed to reflect national health care priorities and views on the most pressing areas for improvement.

Conclusion

Little evidence exists to support one of the above options over another; the committee recognizes that the choice of which system to use involves many value-laden decisions. However, the committee also recognizes that not enough efficiency measures are currently available for this domain to have equal weight with the others, even though efficiency is critical when a payment system is being restructured to reward value. The committee therefore believes option 3 is currently the most viable for an initial pay-for-performance program.

Distribution Between Parts A and B

As described previously, Medicare has different components—Parts A, B, C, and D—that cover and pay for services delivered by different types of providers. Along with how the reward pools for each part are to be developed, distribution to each part must be considered. Once measures have been developed to enable rewards on the basis of episodes or health outcomes, mechanisms will have to be devised for determining the amounts each component should contribute to the reward pool. Similarly, mechanisms will have to be developed for dividing the rewards among all providers who contributed to the high-quality performance. In certain situations, such as inpatient hospital care, that challenge will have to be addressed upon the introduction of any pay-for-performance program because the performance of the hospital will represent the efforts both of the hospital and of physicians and other professionals who are not employees of the hospital. For specific discussion of each of the above settings, see Appendixes A and E.

Payout per Provider

Given the above design issues, this section describes how a provider might expect to be rewarded. The example in Box 4-1 is just one possible method for rewarding physicians based on the principles articulated in this chapter. It assumes that rewards would be allocated based on (1) provider type (e.g., hospital, physician, home health agency), (2) condition, (3) a blended approach rewarding both improvement and excellence, and (4) use of absolute thresholds.

The example in Box 4-1 includes many of the committee's views on how rewards should be distributed. It is important to note that this is a simplified example for ease of understanding; the actual design of payout per provider would be much more nuanced, dealing with multiple physicians treating a single patient's medical condition. The committee believes a pay-for-performance program should not reward providers merely on a per service basis. In the above example, payment is provided per patient per condition. To address the issue of volume (e.g., those physicians treating only 5 diabetics being compared with those treating 20), a standard maximum reward per patient should be paid for each condition. The payment scale described in this example necessarily involves many value-laden decisions. The rate of increase in rewards based on weight does not necessarily have to be linear. The improvement, excellence, and payment scales should all be reassessed periodically and readjusted before each payout to account for changes in performance. This example also focuses only on clinical qual-

BOX 4-1 Example of How a Physician in an Ambulatory Setting Could Be Rewarded on Clinical Quality

Dr. Roller is an internist with approximately 1500 patients, many of whom are covered by Medicare. He treats his Medicare patients for a variety of conditions, including coronary artery disease, chronic heart failure, diabetes, and pneumonia. In this example, Dr. Roller's reward is determined through the calculation of composite scores for selected conditions. Points are assigned for both improvement and excellence. These points are then associated with dollar amounts to create Dr. Roller's total bonus payment.

Composite Score

For his patients with coronary artery disease, Dr. Roller is evaluated by Medicare on how well he performs on the following clinical quality measures: drug therapy for lowering LDL cholesterol, beta-blocker treatment after heart attack, and persistent beta-blocker treatment following myocardial infarction.

These measures (M_{1-3}) are used to form a *composite score* (C_{CAD}). One method, among many for calculating this score, averages the percentages for each measure. Thus if Dr. Roller scores 79 percent, 89 percent, and 71 percent on these three measures, respectively, his composite will be:

$$C_{CAD} = M_1 + M_2 + M_3$$
$$C_{CAD} = (79\% + 89\% + 71\%)/3 = 80\%$$

Measuring Improvement

In the previous year, Dr. Roller's composite score for coronary artery disease was 72 percent. His improvement over the previous year is calculated using the reduction in failure rate (RFR)[*]:

$$RFR = (\text{baseline} - \text{follow-up})/(\text{baseline} - 100\%)$$
$$RFR = (0.72 - 0.8)/(0.72 - 1.0)$$
$$RFR = -0.08/-0.28$$
$$RFR = 0.29 \text{ or } 29\%$$

Rewarding Improvement and Excellence

Dr. Roller's composite score is then compared with thresholds for improvement and excellence for each condition, set by CMS. These points can be combined for a total score. For coronary artery disease, the threshold to be eligible for rewards on improvement could be 20 percent, and the threshold for excellence could be 80 percent. The points achieved for improvement could be scaled:

10% RFR = 0 points	50% RFR = 0.25 points	90% RFR = 0.45 points
20% RFR = 0.10 points	60% RFR = 0.30 points	100% RFR = 0.50 points
30% RFR = 0.15 points	70% RFR = 0.35 points	
40% RFR = 0.20 points	80% RFR = 0.40 points	

For excellence, the following type of scale could be used:

80% = 0.10 points	95% = 0.40 points
85% = 0.20 points	100% = 0.50 points
90% = 0.30 points	

Dr. Roller's points for improvement and excellence are both 0.10. His care of patients with coronary artery disease receives a total of 0.20 points.

Payout

Similar calculations are used for Dr. Roller's patients with diabetes, chronic heart failure, and pneumonia. These composites could be equally weighted and combined in the following manner to determine the overall reward he receives:

$$\text{Payout per provider}_c = \sum(\text{points}_c \times \text{payment}_c),$$
where c = condition, and payment_c = payment scale.

The payment scale should reflect the following considerations:

• Dollar amounts (per patient per condition) should be associated with each weight.
• Rewards should be allocated based on how weights are distributed per condition.

In this system, the provider is rewarded more for each additional patient he sees with a targeted condition.

---

*Reduction in failure rate is the change in performance from baseline to follow-up, divided by the difference between baseline and perfect (100 percent) performance.

ity in the ambulatory setting. Similar models could be developed for rewarding measures of both patient-centeredness and efficiency whereby thresholds would have to be met for a provider to receive rewards for improvement and excellence. Payments in each domain of measures would be aggregated to determine the total amount of a provider's reward. Comparable methods could be developed to award high performance in other care settings, although each setting has unique characteristics that must be accounted for (see Appendix B). Regardless of how pay for performance is designed, it must be transparent and understood by all stakeholders, especially providers and purchasers.

HOW LARGE REWARDS MUST BE

A critical question to be addressed in a pay-for-performance program is how large rewards must be in order to influence provider behavior. There is little evidence regarding the necessary magnitude of rewards (see Chapter 3 for some examples). It is likely that the threshold reward size will vary depending on provider type (e.g., institutional versus individual providers), area of improvement (e.g., conditions, measures, types of improvement interventions), and the percentage of the provider's revenue that is affected by the performance incentives. At the same time, there are constraints in that the amount of the rewards available must be found within Medicare, a program with limited resources. Rewards therefore must be reasonable enough to influence provider behaviors while remaining within the confines of a strict budget. In addition, it is worth noting that payment incentives will be accompanied by public dissemination of performance data, which may prove to be an even more powerful motivator for improving overall quality.

Pay for performance uses incentives to encourage providers to improve. Therefore, if the potential rewards are not large enough to cover the costs associated with improvement, providers may not believe the investment to be worthwhile. If providers are not able to recoup their investment, they may not support the program and decide not to participate (see Chapter 5). By contrast, if the size of rewards is optimized to retain physician buy-in and change provider behaviors, it may offer enough incentive for providers to invest heavily in improving their performance.

SUMMARY

The lack of significant evidence for how an optimal national pay-for-performance program should be designed led the committee to consider many options for distributing rewards to providers. If pay for performance is implemented in Medicare, the committee believes certain principles should apply, such as the importance of rewarding multiple domains of care and the need to reward both improvement and excellence. The design characteristics described in this chapter are general examples that can be adapted to fit the needs of the program with respect to its overarching goals, as defined by CMS.

The next chapter discusses several practical issues to be considered when developing and implementing pay for performance. The committee was able to make firm recommendations on some of these issues, whereas for others, the evidence base supports only careful presentation of options. These issues include the following:

- The timing of pay for performance and its precursors: what steps need to occur before rewards can be provided on the basis of measures of performance.
- The overall timing of implementation: when pay for performance can begin in each care setting.
- The nature of participation: what providers will be eligible for pay for performance in Medicare and whether the program should be voluntary or mandatory.
- The unit of analysis: to whom rewards will be distributed (i.e., the individual physician, medical groups, hospitals, skilled nursing facilities).
- The role of health information technology: how new technologies can influence the implementation of pay for performance.
- Statistical issues: sample size, problems surrounding risk adjustment, and precision.

REFERENCES

Bradley EH, Herrin J, Elbel B, McNamara RL, Magid DJ, Nallamothu BK, Wang Y, Normand S-LT, Spertus JA, Krumholz HM. 2006. Hospital quality for acute myocardial infarction: Correlation among process measures and relationship with short-term mortality. *Journal of the American Medical Association* 296(1):72–78.

IOM (Institute of Medicine). 2001. *Crossing the Quality Chasm: A New Health System for the 21st Century*. Washington, DC: National Academy Press.

IOM. 2006. *Performance Measurement: Accelerating Improvement*. Washington, DC: The National Academies Press.

Jha AK, Li Z, Orav EJ, Epstein AM. 2005. Care in U.S. hospitals: The Hospital Quality Alliance Program. *New England Journal of Medicine* 353(3):265–274.

MedPAC (Medicare Payment Advisory Commission). 2005. *MedPAC Data Runs*. Washington, DC: MedPAC.

5

Implementation

CHAPTER SUMMARY

Chapters 3 and 4 reviewed several alternative methods for creating and distributing a funding pool to reward performance by health care providers who serve Medicare beneficiaries. This chapter addresses major implementation issues that must be considered when new payment schemes designed to create incentives for improved performance by multiple types of health care providers are introduced. This chapter also considers key goals and objectives that should influence the process and pace of implementation of new pay-for-performance programs within different health care environments.

This chapter highlights some procedural and technical issues that might be encountered if a Medicare pay-for-performance program were initially implemented in small steps (such as by care setting or by geographic region) and were subsequently made comprehensive and national in scope:

- Steps in implementing pay for performance and their timing
- The overall timing of implementation
- The nature of participation in payment for performance
- The unit of analysis and reporting
- The role of health information technologies
- Statistical issues

Some lessons can be learned about these issues from existing pay-for-performance efforts, even though many such efforts are still in their infancy. As experience is gained, additional lessons will be learned, and adjustments should be made in Medicare's program accordingly.

STEPS INVOLVED IN IMPLEMENTING PAY FOR PERFORMANCE AND THEIR TIMING

Because a pay-for-perormance program depends on many inputs and the creation of new capabilities, the time needed to implement such a system is an issue that requires careful consideration. Before performance-based rewards can be offered, measures must be developed and tested (as discussed in Chapter 4 and the Institute of Medicine [IOM] report *Performance Measurement: Accelerating Improvement* [IOM, 2006]). Next, data reflecting these measures must be collected and audited, and then distributed to providers for review and feedback. The performance data must then be publicly reported before the final step of paying providers for their performance can be implemented.

Data Collection and Auditing and Provider Feedback

Following the development and testing of performance measures (which as noted was discussed in detail in the *Performance Measurement* report), the next step toward pay for performance is data collection. Data reflecting how well each provider performs on a given metric can generally be gathered from administrative claims, surveys, or medical chart review (in order of the lowest to highest time and cost burden imposed on providers). As discussed in Chapter 4, trade-offs must be made because data relating to the most useful measures are often the most difficult to collect. After being collected, the data need to be audited by an independent body to ensure their validity before they are used to determine relative performance and payment. Data collection and audit may take 6 months even under an aggressive timetable. Once the data have been audited, the results should be shared with providers, each of whom should have the opportunity to provide feedback. Even on a tight timeline, feedback may initially take up to another 6 months to complete. On a less aggressive timetable, these essential steps could initially take up to 2 years. After the first cycle of reporting had been completed, however, the time required for feedback could be reduced to less than 1 month (see Figure 5-1). The entire timeline should be condensed wherever feasible without imposing an undue burden on providers; differences in ability by various provider types should be recognized.

Public Reporting

The committee strongly endorses transparency and accountability in health care to better inform all stakeholders, especially patients, about the performance of the care delivery system. To this end, the committee believes that information reflecting how well health care providers perform on spe-

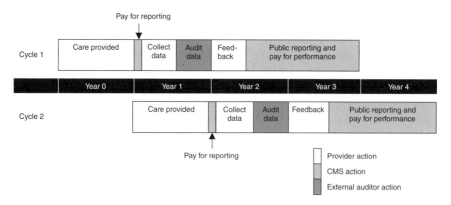

FIGURE 5-1 Example of initial timeline from data collection to pay for performance.

cific measures must be shared with the public and that such public reporting should be a requirement for performance-based payment. Many proponents of public reporting believe this strategy in itself can be a useful tool for improving all aspects of quality, regardless of its association with rewarding performance. To date, the limited evidence presented in the literature is mixed, but overall it does suggest that public reporting can have an impact on provider behaviors and improve quality (Marshall et al., 2000; Hibbard et al., 2005; Jha and Epstein, 2006; Robinowitz and Dudley, 2006).

At the same time, public reporting could have unintended adverse consequences. For example, some providers might avoid sicker patient populations, and others might choose not to participate in Medicare if public reporting on performance became a condition for participation. Notwithstanding the literature that argues otherwise, some low-performing providers might fear that public disclosure of performance data would attract malpractice claims in which the data could be used against them (Werner and Asch, 2005; Kesselheim et al., 2006).

Current Public Reporting Efforts in Medicare

Through the development of the Compare websites by the Centers for Medicare and Medicaid Services (CMS),[1] many providers are already publicly reporting performance data. In 1999, the Medicare Personal Plan

---

[1]CMS has developed a series of websites for the public disclosure of performance data for a variety of providers. Currently available at medicare.gov are Nursing Home Compare, Home Health Compare, Dialysis Facility Compare, Hospital Compare, Medicare Personal Plan Finder (for health plans), and Medicare Prescription Drug Plan Finder.

Finder began comparing the performance of health plans participating in the Medicare+Choice (now Medicare Advantage) program. In 2003, CMS began collecting and reporting data for nursing homes, home health agencies, dialysis facilities, and hospitals. The Medicare Prescription Drug Plan Finder, which allows beneficiaries to compare the premiums and benefits of the various prescription drug plans, was made available in 2005. Beginning in 2006, CMS initiated voluntary reporting for physicians.

Health plans, nursing homes, home health agencies,[2] and dialysis facilities must all report on some services to CMS to receive payments. Reporting is voluntary for hospitals and physicians. In the case of hospitals, however, a small portion of payments—0.4 percent in 2005 and 2 percent in 2006—is withheld from those that do not report as delineated in the Deficit Reduction Act of 2005 (Public Law 109-171); the result has been more than 94 percent of hospitals reporting (CMS, 2006). It is reasonable to suggest that the pay-for-performance approach proposed in this report could be implemented more expeditiously in those settings for which CMS has already been collecting and publicly reporting performance-related data.

Usability

While a number of performance reports from both public and private programs are already available, they are often not particularly helpful to or used by consumers. In the future, not all measures that may be publicly reported to assist consumers will be relevant to pay for performance, and not all measures used in pay for performance will be meaningful to consumers. However, the committee believes that to enhance the integrity of the system, all measures of performance affecting payment should be publicly available. Data must be presented in a fashion that is easy to understand and has meaning for consumers (Hibbard et al., 2000, 2002; Vaiana and McGlynn, 2002). The growing evidence base that explores the types of information and formats the public finds most comprehensible should be consulted to inform public postings. Clearly, as recommended in the *Performance Measurement* report (IOM, 2006), more research is needed to identify the formats most informative for consumers, particularly as the movement toward web-based venues for the presentation of information continues. Multiple reports may need to be developed for different audiences.

Pay for Public Reporting

As noted in Chapter 4, a major area of concern is the magnitude of the burden that might be imposed by data collection, review, and report-

---

[2]All home health agencies are affected, with the exception of hospital-based home health agencies.

ing. The costs associated with collecting and reporting data may be significant, especially for small providers such as independent physicians. A common suggestion for easing the burden of data collection and reporting is the use of health information technologies. As discussed later in this chapter, however, many barriers to the adoption of such technologies exist, including a lack of technical expertise, little agreement on software standards, and cost.

> **Recommendation 6: Because public reporting of performance measures should be an integral component of a pay-for-performance program for Medicare, the Secretary of DHHS should offer incentives to providers for the submission of performance data, and ensure that information pertaining to provider performance is transparent and made public in ways that are both meaningful and understandable to consumers.**

There are two views on how the burden of reporting should be treated. Some argue that the costs associated with collecting and reporting data should be considered a portion of the investment providers must make to be eligible for rewards. Others believe that providers should not be forced to bear these costs until there is convincing evidence that pay for performance can enhance performance and that enhanced performance will lead to significant rewards.

The committee proposes that, initially at least, providers receive payment for collecting, submitting, and reviewing the performance-related data that will be publicly reported and used in the pay-for-perormance program. Financial incentives for the initial submission of data would help defray providers' costs for coding and collecting performance data that cannot be obtained from existing administrative or claims records. Such incentives might also reduce provider opposition to the new system.

The committee believes the pool of funds supporting such incentives should be modest, comparable to those resources used to provide incentives for the voluntary reporting of performance measures by acute care hospitals, and that these payments should end when the collection and reporting of performance measures become routine. Because the committee envisions the continuous development of new and more complex metrics, focused on measures of efficiency and shared accountability, reporting incentives could correspondingly be redirected to new areas that are more complex and difficult to measure. This approach would ensure that providers are not paid merely for the submission of routine data, but are offered incentives that encourage and reward public reporting in areas that can serve as potential levers to improve overall quality. The rewards associated with public reporting should be a small fraction of those devoted to rewarding performance.

Pay for Performance

Only after data have been publicly reported for a predetermined period of time should providers be rewarded based on their performance. This lag time would give providers a chance to become comfortable with the reporting system. Providers would also gain an understanding of how their rewards were derived because during this interim period, CMS would send them estimates of what those rewards would have been had the data affected their payments. Moreover, consumers would have the opportunity to respond to the data by switching providers. Under this timetable, pay for performance based on performance measures available for collection at the start of the program would take place during the second year of implementation (see Figure 5-1). It is important to note that this entire process—from data collection to pay for performance—would be a continuous one. While providers were being rewarded on the basis of old performance data, new data would be collected, distributed, and reported to begin the next cycle of pay for performance. Thus the data used to provide the initial rewards during year 2 would be reflecting performance from year 0 and would have been collected and audited during year 1; data for the next cycle of pay for performance would be reflective of care in year 1 (see Figure 5-1). While rewards initially would be based on data that were 2 years old, over time this lag could be shortened as CMS developed better data collection systems (see the discussion later in this chapter regarding health information technologies) and other strategies.

OVERALL TIMING OF PAY-FOR-PERFORMANCE IMPLEMENTATION

As described in Chapter 4, the committee recommends rewarding providers in three domains—clinical quality, patient-centeredness, and efficiency—as an overarching principle. The committee identified two overall timing options for implementing pay for performance across these three domains. An example of how these options could occur in the ambulatory setting is presented in Box 5-1.

Option 1: Phased Implementation

The first option would be phased implementation, in which pay for performance would begin in each domain as measures became available. Because measures are less developed in some domains than in others, however, there are problems with this approach. For example, the amount distributed from the reward pool would be limited if measures were lacking for one dimension, such as efficiency. Without distribution of the full reward pool, incentives might be inadequate to change provider behavior.

**BOX 5-1   Example of Phased and Delayed Implementation
in the Ambulatory Setting**

In the ambulatory setting, a *phased implementation* could follow the timeline presented below, based on the state of measures in each domain:

	Clinical Quality (AQA measure set)	Patient-Centeredness (Ambulatory CAHPS)	Efficiency
Year 1 (2008)	Collect, audit, gather feedback	Collect, audit, gather feedback	Develop measures
Year 2 (2009)	Public reporting	Public reporting	Pilot test measures
Year 3 (2010)	**Pay for performance**	**Pay for performance**	Collect, audit, gather feedback
Year 4 (2011)	**Pay for performance**	**Pay for performance**	Public reporting

In this example, pay for performance on clinical quality and patient-centeredness would begin in 2010. Pay for reporting (smaller amounts than the rewards for performance) would be implemented in 2008 to help defray the costs of data collection. The collection of these data has begun to some extent through CMS's Physician Voluntary Reporting Program. Rewarding on measures of efficiency would not begin until 2012, with pay for reporting in 2010. However, one option for rewarding on resource use during the intervening period would be to give physicians meeting certain thresholds on both clinical quality and patient-centeredness measures an additional reward if they, by some crude measures, were within the most efficient third of providers. The most efficient

Option 2: Delayed Implementation

The second option would be to delay implementation of pay for performance until a robust set of performance measures had been developed for all three domains. Pay for reporting would begin as measures were developed in each domain and data collection began, but pay for performance would be delayed until after public reporting for all three domains had commenced. If the program's funding mechanism started when performance third of providers could be calculated from standardized costs for Medicare Parts A and B. These costs could be derived from national prices, such as an average payout per unit on the resource-based relative value scale. This method of rewarding efficiency would be phased out upon the development of more sophisticated measures.

In contrast, *delayed implementation* of pay for performance in the ambulatory setting might occur on the following timeline:

	Clinical Quality (AQA measure set)	Patient-Centeredness (Ambulatory CAHPS)	Efficiency
Year 1 (2008)	Collect, audit, gather feedback	Collect, audit, gather feedback	Develop measures
Year 2 (2009)	Public reporting	Public reporting	Pilot test measures
Year 3 (2010)	Public reporting	Public reporting	Collect, audit, gather feedback
Year 4 (2011)	Public reporting	Public reporting	Public reporting
Year 5 (2012)	**Pay for performance**	**Pay for performance**	**Pay for performance**

Under this option, physicians would receive payment for reporting on clinical quality and patient-centeredness measures beginning in 2008. Reporting on efficiency measures would not be rewarded until 2010. Rewards for all three domains on the basis of performance would begin in 2012.

NOTE: AQA = Ambulatory care Quality Alliance; CAHPS = Consumer Assessment of Healthcare Providers and Systems.

measures were being developed and the rewards for reporting were less than collected funds, a larger pool would accumulate for initial performance rewards. This delayed implementation approach would ensure that provider behavior did not overemphasize one domain over the others and that rewards would be distributed only for care that was of high clinical quality, patient-centered, and efficient. The disadvantage of this option is that pay for performance might not begin for many years, and the sense of urgency on this issue might be dissipated.

Conclusion

The committee concludes that phased implementation (option 1) is the preferred approach because it recognizes the urgent need to improve the health care system as quickly as possible. Efforts described in this report to make available a large number of measures of clinical quality and the movement toward better characterizing patient experiences are representative of the momentum in both the public and private sectors that argues for earlier onset of pay for performance. The committee believes this momentum should be captured.

PARTICIPATION IN PAY FOR PERFORMANCE

Two key topics related to participation in pay for performance deserve attention: (1) the nature and pace of the phasing in of payment for performance in different health care settings, and (2) the extent to which participation should be voluntary or mandatory.

Phasing in Participation for Different Settings

Initial Implementation

The committee concurs with MedPAC's rankings for initial participation in pay-for-performance programs: (1) Medicare Advantage plans, (2) dialysis facilities, (3) acute care hospitals, (4) home health agencies, and (5) physician practices (MedPAC, 2005a, 2006). Medicare Advantage plans, dialysis centers, and hospitals are positioned to implement pay for performance now because of the availability of performance measures, the reliability of data, and the fact that the necessary supporting infrastructure is in place. Home health agencies, followed by physicians, would be next to be expected to participate in pay for performance. For an implementation timeline, see Figure 5-2.

Exclusion of Other Providers

The committee believes that eventually, all providers should be included in Medicare's pay-for-performance program. At this time, however, adequate performance measures do not exist for certain institutional providers, such as ambulatory surgical centers, clinical laboratories, rural health clinics, and rehabilitation hospitals, and for certain professionals, including nurse practitioners, occupational therapists, physician assistants, and pharmacists. Once adequate performance measures have been developed, the burden of collecting and reporting on these measures has been made man-

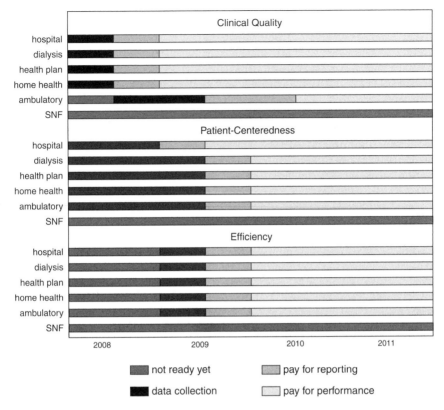

FIGURE 5-2 Implementation timeline for pay for performance.

ageable, and the necessary infrastructure has been put in place, these providers should be brought into the system.

Skilled nursing facilities, not among the institutional providers considered ready for pay for performance as listed in the previous section, deserve special mention. Medicare pays for a specific type of nursing home care provided by these facilities. This specialized care, which represents about one-quarter of all care provided in nursing homes (MedPAC, 2006), follows a medically necessary hospital stay of at least 3 days, is short-term, and is characterized by the use of skilled nursing or rehabilitation services in an inpatient setting.

The committee had several reasons for concluding that it would not be appropriate to reward skilled nursing facilities for performance at this time. First, only 3 of the 15 measures found in the Minimum Data Set—the publicly reported set of measures used to assess nursing home performance—are relevant for short-term stays of the sort paid for by Medicare. Second, these measures (delirium, pain, and pressure ulcers), while important, capture the experiences of only a small portion of beneficiaries covered by Medicare payments to skilled nursing facilities. Third, the data collected do not necessarily capture the quality of care delivered by the facility, as these measures do not accurately reflect the patient's condition upon admission and may reflect care given during the hospital stay (MedPAC, 2005a, 2006). Therefore, the committee concludes that before pay for performance is implemented in skilled nursing facilities, more research is needed to permit better attribution of care. CMS is planning to launch a pay-for-performance demonstration in nursing homes by the end of 2006, which should provide valuable insights for the design of an appropriate pay-for-performance program for nursing homes (The Commonwealth Fund, 2006).

Voluntary Versus Mandatory Participation

Participation in pay for performance may be either voluntary or mandatory. "Participation" involves collecting and submitting to the payer the data needed to construct performance measures, which in turn makes providers eligible to receive financial rewards if they have performed well. With voluntary participation, the individual provider can decide whether to gather and submit performance data and be paid in part on the basis of performance. Under mandatory participation, all providers are required to take part in the system. Mandating participation could burden those providers who would have a difficult time mobilizing the resources required for data collection and reporting, particularly those not closely associated with institutions who may lack access to health information technologies that can ease the burden of those activities. The reliability and validity of data for small providers may also be difficult.

Most private-sector pay-for-performance programs, which tend to focus on physicians, are voluntary. A recent survey of such programs found 91 percent to be voluntary (Baker and Carter, 2005). The propensity toward voluntary programs appears to be related to the heterogeneity of physician practices with respect to their size, specialty focus, location, and use of information technology. Some fear that making such a program mandatory could be too burdensome for certain types of providers, such as small group practices and practices that serve only a handful of a health plan's members. Indeed, programs often differentiate among practices in their requirements for participation. For example, to ensure statistical accuracy, some programs require a minimum volume of patients or a specific ratio of patients treated per physician before a provider is allowed to participate; others permit only providers who have met quality or efficiency thresholds to enroll (Baker and Carter, 2005).

While the experience of the private sector is instructive, several additional considerations are relevant to participation requirements for a Medicare pay-for-performance program. First, Medicare is the provider of primary insurance for virtually all of the elderly and disabled. Therefore, if policy makers want to ensure that all beneficiaries have the opportunity to receive services from providers with incentives to improve all aspects of quality, participation should be mandatory. Second, Medicare beneficiaries constitute a much larger portion of most providers' business than do the members of any single commercial plan, implying that the burden and minimum volume requirements faced by private-sector pay-for-performance programs should be of less concern. Third, as discussed above, many categories of providers already submit performance data to CMS; this is required for some types of providers, voluntary for others, and not expected at all for still others. If all or nearly all providers of a certain type are already submitting the inputs needed for a pay-for-performance program, it would appear sensible to make their participation mandatory. The committee assumes that more measures will be collected in the future for these providers and expects these measures to be incorporated into pay-for-performance programs. Finally, the committee proposes that initial funding of pay for performance be taken out of base payments, which means that the base payments for *all* Medicare providers, whether participating or not, will be reduced to generate resources needed for the incentive reward pool. In the absence of mandatory participation, some providers might argue that they should not have their base payments reduced if they have no chance of being rewarded for good performance (see Figure 5-3).

Option 1: Mandatory Participation

One option for participation in pay for performance is to require that all Medicare providers submit data to CMS for public reporting, and thereby become eligible to receive rewards related to these performance data. Participation would be required as soon as a minimum set of measures was available for each category of provider; those who did not submit the required data to CMS would no longer be considered Medicare providers. Requiring participation could catalyze an accelerated national effort toward performance improvement. While such a stark mandate might be burdensome to CMS, the vast majority of hospitals, home health agencies, dialysis facilities, health plans, and skilled nursing facilities already report some data to CMS that are publicly disclosed. Mandatory participation for physicians and other small providers might be quite challenging if required in the next few years, however.

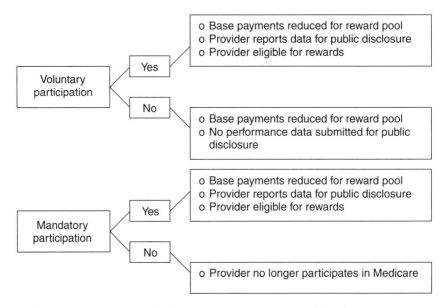

FIGURE 5-3 Outcomes of voluntary and mandatory participation.

Option 2: Voluntary Participation

Allowing providers to choose whether to make the investments neces-sary to participate in pay for performance represents a more cautious ap-proach and one that would engender less stakeholder resistance. While vol-untary participation would be less burdensome to providers who chose not to participate, however, it would undermine the current sense of urgency regarding the need to improve performance and would not capitalize on CMS's public reporting efforts. It is also possible that only those providers who were confident that their performance would be rewarded would join the program, which would do little to raise overall performance. Nonpar-ticipants would argue that their base payments should not be reduced to provide the resources for a program from which they could not benefit.

On the other hand, voluntary participation would reflect some of the underlying realities of the diverse provider community. Many providers have small volumes of Medicare business and have limited capabilities with re-gard to information technologies and data collection and analysis. This is true for some hospitals and other institutional providers, as well as for smaller physician offices. Allowing providers to opt out of a pay-for-performance program, at least until all of the issues involved have been resolved and the effectiveness of the program has been demonstrated, may be a bow to reality.

Option 3: Combination of Mandatory and Voluntary

A third option is to mandate pay for performance among those providers for whom the performance measures and data infrastructure needed to support an incentive-based payment program are available. Providers whose participation could begin immediately with relatively few barriers to implementation are Medicare Advantage plans, dialysis facilities, hospitals, and home health agencies.

Participation for other providers could be phased in when appropriate. Although the necessary measures and data are not yet available for skilled nursing facilities, these providers are already publicly reporting some data to CMS, demonstrating that they do possess the infrastructure necessary for pay for performance. Thus these facilities are in a position to be subject to mandated participation as soon as appropriate measures are available. Measures for other institutional providers, such as clinical laboratories, ambulatory surgical centers, and hospices, are even further behind; the measures are limited, and CMS has not yet developed public reports for these providers. Participation by these other institutions could be mandated given the development of performance measures and positive assessments of these institutions' capabilities to report data publicly.

Many large physician organizations are also ready to participate now in pay for performance. The threshold size of organizations required to participate would be determined by the Secretary of DHHS. Voluntary participation by individual physicians and small physician organizations during the initial phase of pay for performance could improve the acceptance of performance-based rewards by allowing physicians time to develop both confidence in the measures and the structural supports necessary for participation.

Conclusion

The committee recognizes the importance of establishing the expectation that all Medicare providers will participate in public reporting and pay for performance. However, it also recognizes that the pace of implementation, the breadth of measure sets applicable to specific types of providers, and the size and distribution of reward pools will need to vary depending upon the availability of measures and the organizational and technological challenges faced by different providers in carrying out performance measurement and reporting. Efforts should begin immediately to develop and test performance measure sets that fill existing gaps so that all providers can also begin to participate in public reporting and pay for performance as soon as possible.

Some physicians may face greater barriers to implementation than other providers and should therefore be considered separately. CMS should immediately develop and implement a strategy for ensuring that virtually all physicians participate—on at least some measures—as soon as possible. This strategy will need to be sensitive to differences across specialties in the availability of performance measures and the diversity of information systems and operational supports in different practice settings. Financial incentives adequate to ensure early and broad physician participation in the submission of performance measures and public reporting should be employed. Consideration should be given to benefits such as linking accelerated payments or the physician annual payment update to rewards to provide an incentive for public reporting in the same manner that was used with hospitals, as described in the Deficit Reduction Act of 2005. Initial measure sets for pay for performance may need to be limited in some physician settings. In establishing the size of the reward pools, CMS will need to strike a balance between providing financial incentives sizable enough to lead to near-universal participation and recognizing that initial measure sets are narrow, presenting an incomplete picture of a provider's performance.

The transformational changes in the delivery system envisioned in the IOM's *Pathways to Quality Health Care* series of reports will depend upon both the adoption of longitudinal measures of quality that cut across settings and the provision of substantial payment rewards. The strategy used to implement pay for performance should involve moving as soon as practical from the current relatively narrow, provider-specific approach to a more comprehensive, longitudinal set of measures and substantial rewards that encompass all Medicare providers. A monitoring system should be part of the implementation process to inform future decisions about the pace of expansion of the performance measure sets and make it possible to determine whether the voluntary approach initially recommended for physicians is achieving the goal of near-universal participation.

> **Recommendation 7: The Secretary of DHHS should develop and implement a strategy for ensuring that virtually all Medicare providers submit performance measures for public reporting and participate in pay for performance as soon as possible. Initially, measure sets may need to be narrow, but they should evolve over time to provide more comprehensive and longitudinal assessments of provider and system performance. For many institutional providers, participation in public reporting and pay for performance can and should begin immediately. For physicians, a voluntary approach should be pursued initially, relying on financial incentives sufficient to ensure broad participation and recognizing that the**

initial set of measures and the pace of expansion of measure sets will need to be sensitive to the operational challenges faced by providers in small practice settings. Three years after the release of this report, the Secretary of DHHS should determine whether progress toward universal participation is sufficient and whether stronger actions—such as mandating provider participation—are required.

While some small physician organizations and individual physicians are prepared to participate in public reporting and pay-for-performance initiatives, many others will require guidance, technical assistance, and additional infrastructure to make critical transitions in adopting quality procedures and information systems that can enable them to engage in these initiatives. CMS will need to monitor and evaluate the transition phase to identify and share lessons learned at the level of small and individual practices. A target strategy could be used to establish clear goals that could guide this process and to assess progress and unexpected consequences that emerge as pay for performance is phased in over time. Such a strategy could be especially useful for implementation among physicians. In the first phase, for example, only a small percentage of individual physicians or those in practices with only a few physicians might be expected to report data and participate in a performance incentive program. After a year or two, a larger number of physicians might be required to report data to CMS. Another possible target might be for physicians providing more than half of their care to Medicare beneficiaries to submit data and participate in the pay-for-performance program. Performance could also be based initially on a narrow set of measures, preferably ones aligned across public and private payer programs. Physicians could be phased in by the number of areas of specialty care, by the number of states, or by some other selection criteria, as illustrated in Table 5-1. Targets would not be mutually exclusive.

Participation by Specialists

The committee recognizes that specialty care is an integral part of health care: 41.5 percent of visits nationally are made to specialists (NCHS, 2005), and two-thirds of physicians are classified as specialists (U.S. GAO, 2003).[3] Pay-for-performance programs are, however, limited to those providers for whom there are performance measures, and the measures presented in the starter set in Chapter 4 (see Table 4-1) for the most part do not pertain to specialists. The IOM's *Performance Measurement* report found that while

---

[3]Generalists are defined in these two sources as those practicing family and general medicine, internal medicine, and pediatrics. Health, United States also includes those in the field of obstetrics and gynecology.

TABLE 5-1 Illustrative Targets for Phasing in Pay for Performance for Physicians

Year	Physicians (%)	Medicare Beneficiaries as 50% or More of Patient Population (%)	Specialty Areas (number)	States (number)
1	10	100	3	5
2	30	75	10	12
3	50	50	20	25
4	75	30	40	38
5	100	10	60+	50

many measures exist for specialists, such as those developed for thoracic surgeons, these measures need further vetting before being considered robust enough to be used at the national level for payment based on performance (USPSTF, 2006). The lack of specialist measures is a critical gap in performance measures. As mentioned in Chapter 3, pay for performance could help specialists and others accelerate the development of performance measures. Efforts should be made to ensure that newly developed measures are subject to equally rigorous testing for reliability and validity. The committee concludes that measures for specialists should be addressed with the utmost urgency and, once available, be included in pay-for-performance programs.

UNIT OF ANALYSIS AND REPORTING

In designing a pay-for-performance program, it is necessary to decide whether performance measures will be collected for and rewards paid to individual providers or groups of providers who together are responsible for a patient's care. As discussed in Chapter 4, the committee believes it to be unavoidable that rewards will be distributed initially by setting of care. In other words, rewards will be distributed to health plans, dialysis facilities, hospitals, home health agencies, skilled nursing facilities, and physician offices. Ultimately, the committee envisions that performance will be measured by following patients across time and across the various settings in which a patient receives care (see Chapter 2).

Implementation will be different for various types of providers. The unit of analysis for most institutional settings has already been defined as the facility itself, rendering the question of payment being made to individuals or groups of little consequence. On the other hand, rewarding physicians paid under Part B becomes complicated (see Box 5-2).

Virtual Groups

In identifying options for the unit of analysis for physicians, the committee discussed the merits of encouraging the formation of "virtual groups"—groups of physicians who, while not formally connected, would choose to associate with each other in informal ways to promote coordination of care and improve efficiency. This could occur, for example, through patient-determined groups or coordinated use of information technologies. Box 5-3 provides examples of how virtual groups could function to accelerate improvements in care delivery.

Several arguments can be made for encouraging virtual groups. First, performance measures for groups, whether organized or virtual, would be more accurate than those for single physicians or small group practices because the sample sizes would be larger. Second, the ability to compare and discuss clinical quality and efficiency with a number of like-minded providers and possibly share information technology tools could serve to improve overall quality. Third, multispecialty virtual groups could encourage coordination and help overcome the quality deficiencies that arise from poor care coordination among the various physicians treating a single patient.

Many questions need to be addressed in assessing the feasibility of virtual groups. For example, what financial relationships would be required among members? What would the legal structure look like? What would the mechanism be for entering and exiting the group? How could one monitor the impacts as well as the unintended consequences of virtual groups? What would it take to create such groups? Although many such questions must be addressed, the committee supports exploration of the formation of virtual groups.

Promoting Coordination

Health care is often the product of many actors, as patients tend to be treated by more than a single provider. On average, Medicare beneficiaries are treated by 5 physicians during a year. Those with such chronic conditions as chronic heart failure, coronary artery disease, and diabetes see an average of 13 different physicians in a year (MedPAC, 2005b). Patients are also treated in multiple care settings, moving, for example, among physician offices, hospitals, and long-term care facilities. As discussed in Chapter 2, the health care received by Medicare beneficiaries is often fragmented and not well coordinated. This critical problem is thought to result in worse

---

**BOX 5-2   Example of Units of Analysis
in the Ambulatory Setting**

Physician offices differ from other settings in part because of issues of sample size. The literature has shown that for measures to represent adequately how well providers are performing, on average 25 cases are needed (personal communication, G. Pawlson, August 3, 2006). Since the committee argues that rewards should be linked directly to how well providers perform based on a composite score for a specific condition (see Chapter 4), a physician would have to see a minimum of 25 patients per condition, referred to as cases, to be eligible for rewards. However, a single primary care physician may not see 25 or more asthmatics or diabetics, and a physician who did not have a sufficient number of cases would not qualify for rewards for that condition. This issue also raises the question of whether rewards will be large enough to be financially meaningful to providers. To address these issues, the committee examined three alternatives for providing rewards at the physician office level.

Option 1: Individual Physicians. Under this option, individual physicians with sufficient numbers of cases would be eligible for rewards associated with performance. The care attributable to each physician would be known and could therefore be rewarded appropriately. Because care would be attributable to individual physicians, a shared sense of responsibility could result from this option. However, many physicians do not see enough patients for measures to be reliable, and it is difficult to estimate resource use. Moreover, rewards may be too small under this option for physicians to seriously consider participating in pay for performance. This option also poses the technical problem of attributing patients to physicians (Pham, 2006).

---

health outcomes. One way to address this problem is to provide direct and indirect incentives for care coordination. To the extent that pay for performance rewards specific providers for performing at a desired level and care coordination contributes to high-quality care, pay for performance should indirectly encourage better care coordination. Nonetheless, the fragmented nature of care, the increased specialization among professionals, and the inherent difficulty of assigning responsibility for health outcomes may mean that more direct incentives are needed to generate the optimal amount of coordination. To this end, the committee recommends that Medicare encourage beneficiaries and their providers to identify a responsible or accountable source of care. This accountable source of care could take various forms, including (1) the beneficiary's predominant caregiver (e.g., a primary care doctor, a specialist treating a chronic condition), who would agree to be responsible for the coordination of all of the beneficiary's care;

Option 2: Physician Groups. Under this option, rewards for performance would be determined on the basis of the performance of groups of physicians. The group would be responsible for distributing the rewards, allowing for such options as investing some of the money in operational costs. There are advantages to this approach. For example, it would allow physicians to aggregate cases, addressing the issues of sample size and reward size that arise under option 1. Team-oriented care and shared accountability would also be promoted. Finally, rewarding groups could mitigate concerns about public reporting and the stigma of poor performance that arise in measuring the performance of and rewarding individual physicians. Therefore, this option may also enable more rapid implementation of a pay-for-performance program. A disadvantage of this option, however, is that holding specific providers responsible for the care of specific patients would be difficult. The distribution of rewards would be complicated, but this would be an issue for groups themselves to address. Another disadvantage of distributing rewards at the group level is that there is currently a disparity in clinical quality between care delivered by individual and small-practice physicians as compared with large physician groups (Bodenheimer et al., 2005). This method would likely increase that gap.

Option 3: Combination of Options 1 and 2. This option would initially reward physician groups until measures that could reliably assess care at the individual physician level were available. Physicians would be allowed to opt to be rewarded at either level during the transition to the long-term approach of using individuals as the unit of analysis.

(2) an advanced medical home;[4] or (3) an integrated health care system. The responsible source of care would be accountable for the attribution of care delivered by the beneficiary's various providers, as well as for the patient's improved outcomes, safety, and efficiency. Being accountable for the patient would include being in charge of guiding the patient through the complex health care system, making referrals, checking for contraindicated medications, and having an integrated medical record with a complete medical history. The responsible source of care should be compensated for serving this function.

---

[4]The definition used here has been modified to refer to multiple primary care practices linked through information technology systems that pool resources to support the structural capabilities needed to provide a coordinating function. Such structural capabilities include having nurse educators and dieticians. The term was originally developed by the American College of Physicians (ACP, 2006).

Recommendation 8: The Centers for Medicare and Medicaid Services (CMS) should design the Medicare pay-for-performance program to include components that promote, recognize, and reward improved coordination of care across providers and through entire episodes of illness. Thus, CMS should (1) encourage beneficiaries and providers to identify providers who would be considered their principal responsible source of care, and (2) pay for and reward successful care coordination that meets specified standards for providers who take on that role.

BOX 5-3   Examples of Virtual Groups

Example 1: Hospitalization-Related Virtual Group

A virtual group could be defined as the hospital medical staff and physicians caring for all patients admitted for a particular condition. For example, all patients admitted to hospital A for acute myocardial infarction during a given year could be identified as the study population. All physicians who provided any care for 25 or more of these patients during the year following their index admission would be identified as part of the virtual group and eligible for inclusion in the incentive system. Quality would be assessed using the best currently available measures, including, presumably, risk-adjusted 1-year survival and adherence to the Hospital Quality Alliance and the Ambulatory care Quality Alliance technical quality measures. Resource use would be measured using price-standardized measures (e.g., relative value units, diagnosis-related groups, nursing home per diems) and would include all care received by these patients, regardless of where it was provided (including out of the area). Performance could be compared with that of similar groups or with the group's own performance during the prior year. Rewards for improved quality and efficiency could be allocated within the virtual group based on the proportion of evaluation and management claims for services provided to the cohort. The group could also be expanded to include other cohorts (cancer, orthopedics) to increase the number of physicians involved in the reward system.

Example 2: Horizontal Virtual Group

Ten independent primary care physicians located in the same geographic area could agree to create a virtual group to foster a care management process for their patients with chronic conditions, which could

It must be recognized that not all providers treating Medicare beneficiaries would be willing or able to serve this coordinating function. The Secretary of DHHS should design the particulars of how providers would be rewarded for serving this function, in addition to being eligible for rewards based on performance. The funding for this purpose need not come from the pay-for-performance reward pools discussed in Chapter 3, but could be drawn from the basic payment systems within Medicare.

Beneficiaries would have an important role in this process, in that they would work with their providers to identify a responsible source of care.

improve quality and value while reducing overall costs. These physicians might jointly purchase an electronic health information system, as well as discuss guidelines and the evidence base for best care practices at a monthly meeting. In joining this virtual group, the ten physicians would agree to share the costs associated with purchase and implementation of the electronic system as well as training in its use. In addition, the virtual group might agree to share the costs and administration of enhanced clinical support, such as the following:

- Nurses who would serve as care managers for high-risk patients and visit patients living with targeted chronic conditions for all ten physicians.
- Bidirectional data provided by a common laboratory vendor to reduce data entry costs.
- "Service agreements" negotiated with an identified group of specialists who agreed to use methods approved by all the physicians and increase communication between primary and secondary care providers.

Example 3: Virtual Groups Convened by Health Plans

Health plans could play a convening role in the formation of virtual groups, for example, by providing a common information technology platform for gathering data across multiple solo or small group practices in return for a small fee. Practices would not have to be located in the same geographic area, as they would be linked by common financial and communication systems. As part of their services, plans could also track a minimum number of patients with chronic conditions and send out prompts and reminders for recommended preventive services. Reward sharing could occur through reaching of thresholds on selected performance measures (including clinical effectiveness and efficiency) for chronic conditions determined by CMS.

Incentives, such as reductions in Medicare Part B premiums, could be used to encourage beneficiaries to make this designation. The mechanisms for this involvement should be easy for beneficiaries to understand and apply. Moreover, all activities related to this process should protect patient confidentiality and be completed in compliance with the regulations of the Health Insurance Portability and Accountability Act.

The committee recognizes the many technical difficulties associated with implementing such a process. Nonetheless, the committee believes enhancing care coordination is essential to improving the overall quality of care and should be promoted through the use of incentives to the extent possible.

THE ROLE OF HEALTH INFORMATION TECHNOLOGIES

Potential Benefits

Information technologies might be used as a transformative tool in systems change to enhance health care delivery. For example, computerized provider order entry systems can help minimize errors in prescribing medications. Electronic health records can facilitate clinical documentation and potentially allow providers to have more complete and comprehensive information about their patients available at the point of care, and can enable improvements in the safety, effectiveness, and efficiency of treatment by making a patient's medical records portable among multiple providers.

With respect to pay for performance, health information technologies can assist providers in data collection and reporting activities. Although the evidence is limited, use of these technologies may reduce the burden on providers and their staffs associated with reviewing medical records for reporting purposes as the number of measures grows, improve the accuracy of the data reported, and expedite the implementation of pay for performance. The sooner data are received and validated, the sooner rewards can be determined and distributed to providers. It is also true that pay for performance can encourage adoption of information technologies. If information technologies are indeed found to greatly facilitate improvement, their adoption may increase significantly. The following discussion assesses the current state of adoption, current activities, and barriers to implementation of health information technologies.

Current State of Adoption

Despite the potential importance of health information technologies, their adoption has been slow in both inpatient and ambulatory settings, with most efforts having been initiated in the private sector. Several surveys of physician practices have found that less than one-third of physicians (12–27 percent) use electronic health records (Anderson et al., 2005; Heffler et al., 2005; Reed and Grossman, 2006; Safran et al., 2006). Moreover, only a small proportion of the electronic health records used by ambulatory care practices possess the capabilities, including basic decision support (e.g., drug interaction alerts, notification of abnormal test results) needed to improve efficiency and quality (Heffler et al., 2005; Reed and Grossman, 2006). The extent to which electronic health records are actually designed to facilitate public reporting, however, remains unclear.

In larger, more complex health care settings, such as hospitals and health care systems, the most successful electronic health records tend to be the result of systems built in stages over many years (Chaudhry et al., 2006). Larger hospitals also tend to have higher information technology usage rates than smaller hospitals (Felt-Lisk, 2006). As of 2005, many hospitals (approximately 50 percent) had automated their major ancillary clinical systems (i.e., pharmacy, laboratory, radiology) and were incorporating those data into clinical data repositories that allow for physician access to review and retrieve results (Schoen et al., 2005). However, very few hospitals have implemented either sophisticated electronic systems capable of clinical documentation and decision support (approximately 8 percent) or computerized provider order entry that is available to any clinician (2–6 percent) (Berwick, 2002; Schoen et al., 2005). Moreover, the use of information technologies in hospitals has not yet significantly improved the quality of public reporting (Felt-Lisk, 2006).

Electronic systems should not be the same for all providers, as different providers have different needs. For example, computerized provider order entry systems in hospitals include capabilities for laboratory, radiology, and consults; none of these services are necessary for a system designed to be used in a skilled nursing facility. Adoption rates also tend to differ by provider size. According to one study, smaller providers (i.e., home health agencies, skilled nursing facilities, and groups of fewer than five physicians) can be expected to have less well-developed electronic capabilities than larger groups (i.e., hospitals and groups of 20 or more physicians), probably because of limited financial and personnel resources (Kaushal et al., 2005).

Current Activities

The federal government has initiated activities to support the development of health information technologies, as will be underscored by an executive order from the Bush Administration to require all federally financed providers to adopt uniform information technology standards and quality measurement tools (Broder, 2006). Primary among these activities is development of a National Health Information Network (NHIN) through several efforts, including the following:

- The Consolidated Health Informatics (CHI) initiative, which has endorsed a portfolio of existing health information interoperability standards (Bodenheimer, 2005).
- The Healthcare Information Technology Standards Panel, a cooperative partnership of public and private stakeholders, supported and funded by the DHHS Office of the National Coordinator for Health Information Technology with the purpose of achieving a widely accepted and useful set of standards that will enable and support widespread interoperability among health care software applications (ANSI, 2006).
- The American Health Information Community, a commission of public and private representatives that provides input and recommendations to DHHS on the development and adoption of architecture, standards, a certification process, and a method of governance for the ongoing implementation of health information technology (Thorpe, 2005).
- A set of 16 community health information technology grants totaling more than $22.3 million, awarded by the Agency for Healthcare Research and Quality (AHRQ), which are focused on data sharing and interoperability among providers, laboratories, pharmacies, and patients in several regions across the country (Cogan et al., 2005).
- Contracts totaling $18.6 million awarded by DHHS to four consortia of technology developers and health care providers to develop prototypes for an NHIN (Dowd, 2005); and
- Partial or full funding in support of more than 100 Regional Health Information Organizations (RHIOs)—regional collaborations throughout the country that facilitate the development, implementation, and application of secure health information systems across care settings (including those funded by AHRQ as noted above) (Ginsburg, 2005).

In addition, in the private sector, Connecting for Health has begun a National Health Information Exchange initiative, which involves three very different local health information networks—in Boston, Massachusetts; Indianapolis, Indiana; and Mendocino, California—that will work together to facilitate their secure exchange of health information (Rosenthal et al., 2005). Several RHIOs are also under way that are fully supported by private industries and/or state legislation. The federal government and other public and private stakeholders need to continue to work aggressively on the development of these mechanisms for interoperability among health information technology systems, while also ensuring the confidentiality of individual patient information.

Barriers to Implementation

The extent to which health information technologies can yield savings or better health outcomes is unclear. Gains have been proven only in large health systems and after long implementation processes. The current low level of adoption of health information technology is due to many challenges, not the least of which is cost. Electronic health record systems are an expensive and high-risk investment—one that involves not only initial acquisition and implementation costs, but also the more significant costs of short-term productivity loss, ongoing training, redesign of clinical and administrative processes, and the process of changing the way work is performed.

The issue of cost was also complicated by the existence of certain federal laws (i.e., the physician self-referral law ["Stark Law"] and the anti-kickback statute) intended to prevent payments to clinicians that might encourage overutilization of health care services. These laws, however, also created barriers to the provision of financial and other assistance by larger to smaller health care providers. On August 1, 2006, the Secretary of DHHS issued two regulations addressing these laws, lifting some of these barriers. Whether the regulations will in fact help accelerate adoption of health information technologies remains to be seen (U.S. DHHS, 2006a,b).

There is also a paucity of quantifiable data in the literature on financial returns on investment in electronic health record systems (Chaudhry et al., 2006). For ambulatory practices, the evidence is beginning to point to positive returns within 3 years, especially when the electronic health record system is integrated with a practice management system, as a result of the cost savings from reduced transcriptions and revenue gains from more appropriate coding (Lied and Sheingold, 2001; Trivedi et al., 2005; Vaccarino et al., 2005). However, electronic health record systems currently are limited in their ability to effectively recall, collate, and analyze data. Evidence regarding the possible benefits of interoperability—the ability to exchange data across providers, sites, and organizations—has been both limited and mixed. Some studies have shown significant cost savings (an annual net value of $113.9–220.9 billion, assuming a 15-year adoption period) (Moran, 2005), while others have found none. In addition, while the federal government and others have made some progress in the promulgation of national standards for health care information exchange and interoperability—through the foundational work of the CHI initiative and the ongoing work of the Healthcare Information Technology Standards Panel, the American Health Information Community, and RHIOs—there is still a long way to go.

Another challenge faced by physician practices and hospitals has been the lack of guidance for selecting and implementing electronic health record systems; it is difficult to know whether a given system will provide the necessary functionality in both the short and long terms and whether the vendor will remain in business to provide upgrades and ongoing technical assistance. Several efforts have been initiated to address this issue. DHHS has commissioned the Certification Commission for Healthcare Information Technology, a private, nonprofit organization, to develop and evaluate the certification criteria and inspection process for electronic health record systems. In addition, many public- and private-sector stakeholders—including CMS (through its Doctor's Office Quality-Information Technology program), Medicare (through its Quality Improvement Organizations), professional organizations, trade associations, and industry websites—are beginning to offer technical assistance to both hospitals and physicians.

Finally, both clinicians and consumers have demonstrated resistance to the adoption of electronic health record systems to aid in systems changes. It is often thought that clinicians will need to adopt a fundamentally different way of making and documenting clinical decisions to incorporate electronic health records into their practices. The initial phase of implementation, in particular, will result in longer work hours for clinicians as they become familiar with the application and enter background information for each patient (Trivedi et al., 2005). In addition, decision supports are more useful if the input data are structured and coded, which requires that clinicians use structured input supports, such as checklists. Consumers are also resistant because of concerns about the privacy and confidentiality of their records, and physician practices and hospitals are sensitive to these concerns.

Role of Health Information Technologies in Pay for Performance

The adoption of health information technologies could facilitate data collection and reporting, and thereby expedite pay for performance. Although pay for performance might conversely accelerate adoption of information technologies, the committee does not suggest that pay for performance be contingent on providers adopting these technologies. The possession of advanced information systems can place some providers at greater advantage relative to other providers without these capabilities. The committee therefore supports all initiatives in both the public and private sectors to advance the state of health information technology, as well as all research aimed at determining whether and how significant savings associated with electronic systems can be achieved.

Recommendation 9: Because electronic health information technology will increase the probability of a successful pay-for-performance program, the Secretary of DHHS should explore a variety of approaches for assisting providers in the implementation of electronic data collection and reporting systems to strengthen the use of consistent performance measures.

STATISTICAL ISSUES

The validity and acceptability of a system for rewarding performance depends on the quality of the data used to construct the performance measures. To ensure high-quality data, statistical reliability and validity are essential. Implementation of pay for performance also depends on the comparability of data. Appropriate adjustments must be made to the raw data to correct for clear biases and confounding elements that may be beyond the control of the provider. It is important to recognize the major role of beneficiary behavior in overall health care outcomes. These behaviors must be adjusted for and taken into account when the care delivered is being attributed to the performance of individual physicians, especially with respect to outcomes.

Deriving an accurate representation of a provider's performance necessitates meeting minimum requirements for sample size. Sample size refers to the number of cases being used to calculate a measure. If there are not enough cases, poor or excellent outcomes may reflect sample variability rather than true performance. This issue is particularly important with respect to physicians. As noted earlier, many general practitioners may not see 25 patients—viewed as a minimum threshold for performance measures—afflicted with the same condition.

For some measures, the data may be skewed by characteristics of the patient or the environment. For example, a provider's performance measures may look mediocre not because his skills or processes are poor, but because the cases treated are more complex than average or his patients have many comorbidities. Risk adjustment is an attempt to correct for such confounding conditions. Similar adjustments may be necessary for social, cultural, and economic differences in providers' patients. For example, some providers may serve disproportionate numbers of nonadherent patients, patients who are economically disadvantaged and lack supplemental insurance, or those who are unable to communicate effectively with the provider. A pay-for-performance program should not penalize providers who serve such beneficiaries or create incentives to avoid them, recognizing that programs to promote better behavior should be rewarded. Such unintended adverse consequences should be compensated for and should not be neglected. These statistical issues are inherent in performance measurement, but can be adjusted for to better characterize the care that is delivered. However, much research must be completed before an optimal system is available. Methods of better accounting for sample-size problems and carrying out risk adjustment must be formulated to ensure the integrity of a pay-for-performance program.

SUMMARY

Implementation of a pay-for-performance program is complicated. Providers are at different levels of readiness to participate in such a program because of variations in the availability of performance measures and supporting infrastructure. Public reporting is a necessary step in rewarding performance. To help ease the burden of data collection, CMS should pay providers for reporting. It is expected that eventually, all Medicare providers will be rewarded based on their performance. Adequate financial incentives and assistance should be provided to achieve this goal. While information technologies can be useful in accelerating implementation, they are not necessary for success. A pay-for-performance program should be a learning system and should therefore undergo regular comprehensive evaluation. The next chapter addresses monitoring, evaluation, and the research agenda that must be carried out to better understand the effects of pay for performance and optimal future directions.

REFERENCES

ACP (American College of Physicians). 2006. *The Advanced Medical Home: A Patient-Centered, Physician-Guided Model of Health Care*. Philadelphia, PA: ACP.

Anderson GF, Hussey PS, Frogner BK, Waters HR. 2005. Health spending in the United States and the rest of the industrialized world. *Health Affairs* 24(4):903–914.

ANSI (American National Standards Institute). 2006. *Healthcare Information Technology Standards Panel*. [Online]. Available: http://www.htsip.org [accessed May 30, 2006].

Baker G, Carter B. 2005. *Provider Pay-for-Performance Incentive Programs: 2004 National Study Results*. San Francisco, CA: Med-Vantage, Inc.

Berwick D. 2002. A user's manual for the IOM's "Quality Chasm" report. *Health Affairs* 21(3):80–90.

Bodenheimer T. 2005. The political divide in health care: A liberal perspective. *Health Affairs* 24(6):1426–1435.

Bodenheimer T, May JH, Berenson RA, Coughlan J. 2005. *Can Money Buy Quality? Physician Response to Pay for Performance*. Washington, DC: Center for Studying Health System Change.

Broder D. 2006, August 6. Administration aims to set health-care standards. *Washington Post*.

Chaudhry B, Wang J, Wu S, Maglione M, Mojica W, Roth E, Morton SC, Shekelle PG. 2006. Systematic review: Impact of health information technology on quality, efficiency, and costs of medical care. *Annals of Internal Medicine* 144(10):742–752.

CMS (Centers for Medicare and Medicaid Services). 2006. *Hospital Compare*. [Online]. Available: http://www.hospitalcompare.hhs.gov [accessed May 15, 2006].

Cogan JF, Hubbard RG, Kessler DP. 2005. Making markets work: Five steps to a better health care system. *Health Affairs* 24(6):1447–1457.

The Commonwealth Fund. 2006. *Washington Health Policy Week in Review.* [Online]. Available: http://www.cmwf.org/healthpolicyweek/healthpolicyweek_show.htm?doc_id=362624&#doc362626 [accessed June 2, 2006].

Dowd B. 2005. Coordinated agency versus autonomous consumers in health services markets. *Health Affairs* 24(6):1501–1511.

Felt-Lisk S. 2006. *Issue Brief: New Hospital Information Technology: Is It Helping to Improve Quality?* Washington, DC: Mathematica Policy Research, Inc.

Ginsburg P. 2005. Competition in health care: Its evolution over the past decade. *Health Affairs* 24(6):1512–1522.

Heffler S, Smith S, Keehan S, Borger C, Clemens MK, Truffer C. 2005. Trends: U.S. health spending projections for 2004–2014. *Health Affairs* w5.74.

Hibbard JH, Slovic P, Peters E, Finucane M. 2000. *Older Consumers' Skill in Using Comparative Data to Inform Health Plan Choice: A Preliminary Assessment.* Washington, DC: Public Policy Institute, AARP.

Hibbard JH, Slovic P, Peters E, Finucane ML. 2002. Strategies for reporting health plan performance information to consumers: Evidence from controlled studies. *Health Services Research* 37(2):291–313.

Hibbard JH, Stockard J, Tusler M. 2005. Hospital performance reports: Impact on quality, market, share, and reputation. *Health Affairs* 1150–1160.

IOM (Institute of Medicine). 2006. *Performance Measurement: Accelerating Improvement.* Washington, DC: The National Academies Press.

Jha AK, Epstein AM. 2006. The predictive accuracy of the New York state coronary artery bypass surgery report-card system. *Health Affairs* 25(3):844–855.

Kaushal R, Bates DW, Poon EG, Jha AK, Blumenthal D, Harvard Interfaculty Program for Health Systems Improvement NHIN Working Group. 2005. Functional gaps in attaining a national health information network. *Health Affairs* 24(5):1281–1289.

Kesselheim AS, Ferris TG, Studdert DM. 2006. Will physician-level measures of clinical performance be used in medical malpractice litigation? *Journal of the American Medical Association* 295(15):1831–1834.

Lied TR, Sheingold S. 2001. HEDIS performance trends in Medicare managed care. *Health Care Financing Review* 23(1):149–160.

Marshall MN, Shekelle PG, Leatherman S, Brook RH. 2000. The release of performance data: What do we expect to gain? A review of the evidence. *Journal of the American Medical Association* 283(14):1866–1874.

MedPAC (Medicare Payment Advisory Commission). 2005a. *Report to the Congress: Medicare Payment Policy.* Washington, DC: MedPAC.

MedPAC. 2005b. *MedPAC Data Runs.* Washington, DC: MedPAC.

MedPAC. 2006. *Report to the Congress: Medicare Payment Policy.* Washington, DC: MedPAC.

Moran DW. 2005. Whence and whither health insurance? A revisionist history. *Health Affairs* 24(6):1415–1425.

NCHS (National Center for Health Statistics). 2005. *Health, United States, 2005: With Chartbook Trends in the Health of Americans.* Hyattsville, MD: U.S. Government Printing Office.

Pham M. 2006. *How Many Doctors Does It Take to Treat a Patient? The Challenges That Fragmented Care Poses for P4P.* Unpublished.

Reed MC, Grossman JM. 2006. *Data Bulletin: Growing Availability of Clinical Information Technology in Physician Practices.* Washington, DC: Center for Studying Health System Change.

Robinowitz DL, Dudley RA. 2006. Public reporting of provider performance: Can its impact be made greater? *Annual Review of Public Health* 27:517–536.

Rosenthal MB, Frank RG, Li Z, Epstein AM. 2005. Early experience with pay-for-performance: From concept to practice. *Journal of the American Medical Association* 294(14):1788–1793.

Safran DG, Miller W, Beckman H. 2006. Organizational dimensions of relationship-centered care: Theory, evidence, and practice. *Journal of General Internal Medicine* 21(s1): S9–S15.

Schoen C, Osborn R, Huynh PT, Doty M, Zapert K, Peugh J, Davis K. 2005. Taking the pulse of health care systems: Experiences of patients with health problems in six countries. *Health Affairs* w5.509.

Thorpe KE. 2005. The rise in health care spending and what to do about it. *Health Affairs* 24(6):1436–1445.

Trivedi AN, Zaslavsky AM, Schneider EC, Ayanian JZ. 2005. Trends in the quality of care and racial disparities in Medicare managed care. *New England Journal of Medicine* 353(7):692–700.

U.S. DHHS (United States Department of Health and Human Services). 2006a. Medicare and state health care programs: Fraud and abuse; safe harbors for certain electronic prescribing and electronic health records arrangements under the anti-kickback statute; final rule. *Federal Register* 71(152):45109–45137.

U.S. DHHS. 2006b. Medicare program; physicians referrals to health care entities with which they have financial relationships; exceptions for certain electronic prescribing and electronic health records arrangements. *Federal Register* 71(152):45139–45171.

U.S. GAO (United States General Accounting Office). 2003. *Physician Workforce: Physician Supply Increased in Metropolitan and Nonmetropolitan Areas but Geographic Disparities Persisted.* [Online]. Available: http://www.gao.gov/new.items/d04124.pdf [accessed January 12, 2006].

USPSTF (U.S. Preventive Services Task Force). 2006. *Guide to Clinical Preventive Services.* [Online]. Available: http://www.ahrq.gov/clinic/cps.3dix.htm [accessed June 13, 2006].

Vaccarino V, Rathore SS, Wenger NK, Frederick PD, Abramson JL, Barron HV, Manhapra A, Mallik S, Krumholz HM, National Registry of Myocardial Infarction Investigators. 2005. Sex and racial differences in the management of acute myocardial infarction, 1994 through 2002. *New England Journal of Medicine* 353(7):671–682.

Vaiana ME, McGlynn EA. 2002. What cognitive science tells us about the design of reports for consumers. *Medical Care Research and Review* 59(1):35–59.

Werner RM, Asch DA. 2005. The unintended consequences of publicly reporting quality information. *Journal of the American Medical Association* 293(10):1239–1244.

6

Monitoring, Evaluation, and Research: Future Directions

CHAPTER SUMMARY

Pay for performance is one important means by which reimbursement mechanisms can be realigned to promote quality health care. Given both its considerable potential to impact care and the limited experience to date with implementation of such a program, a pay-for-performance program in Medicare should be closely monitored and evaluated so its design and use can quickly be modified to reflect experience gained in the real world. In addition, traditional forms of research must be used to address more technical questions. This chapter presents both a process for ongoing monitoring and evaluation and a research agenda.

Monitoring, evaluation, and research are integral components of a pay-for-performance program and should encompass the following:

- Use of data collected from existing measures to help analyze the effect of pay for performance.
- Processes for developing valid, robust performance measures that are increasingly linked to meaningful clinical outcomes and characterize performance comprehensively.
- The ability to develop real-time monitoring systems that are capable of quickly identifying benefits—both intended and serendipitous—as well as unintended adverse consequences.
- Definition of an initial research agenda to address technical matters pertaining to questions raised in this report.

Monitoring, evaluation, and research functions should not be divorced from program design and implementation or merely appended to pay-for-performance programs. Rather, their success depends on having a strong learning system that is intrinsic to the design and activities of the program. Such a learning system would build on previous experiences and enable Medicare to better fulfill its congressional mandate to serve beneficiaries. In addition, it is expected that the private sector would closely attend to the Medicare experience, supporting the government's mission to articulate national goals and leveraging private resources in concert with the public program. Conversely, the absence of a scientifically valid, comprehensive, integrated, and flexible system—one that facilitated learning from experience—would likely contribute to the failure of a pay-for-performance program. Aggressive actions are necessary now to take full advantage of the opportunity offered by pay for performance by increasing the knowledge base regarding the nexus of reimbursement, provider behavior, and quality of health care.

> **Recommendation 10: The Secretary of DHHS should implement a monitoring and evaluation system for the Medicare pay-for-performance program in order to:**
>
> - Assess early experiences with implementation so timely corrective action can be taken.
> - Evaluate the overall impact of pay for performance on clinical quality, patient-centeredness, and efficiency.
> - Identify the best practices of high-performing delivery settings that should be shared with others to improve care throughout the nation.

This active learning system should be complemented by the identification of a more conventional research agenda through consensus among the major stakeholders and at the national level. This research agenda should address identified gaps in payment methodologies and the incorporation of new measures, and create the context for future investigations as actual experience with pay for performance raises new questions.

FUNDAMENTALS OF EVALUATION AND RESEARCH

Performance measures will be used to evaluate the benefits of pay for performance and to identify the effects of its implementation on health outcomes. Ideal measures should have the following characteristics:

- Pertain to the domains of interest—clinical quality, patient-centeredness, and efficiency.
- Link to meaningful clinical outcomes.
- Be clearly defined.
- Be easily implemented.

The first report in the Institute of Medicine's (IOM's) *Pathways* series—*Performance Measurement: Accelerating Improvement*—identified measures of potential value as well as gaps in existing measures to be filled through directed research (IOM, 2006b). The second report in the series—*Medicare's Quality Improvement Organization Program: Maximizing Potential*—emphasized the need for expert technical assistance to providers attempting to use performance measurement for quality improvement purposes (IOM, 2006a). Performance measurement requires attention to the integrity and validity of baseline assessments so the impact of aligning reimbursement mechanisms through pay for performance can be accurately assessed. Performance measures pertinent to pay for performance should have clear metrics that are easy to interpret and implement; the burden on providers associated with the collection of the data should be reasonable; and the results should be clearly presented and easy to understand by all consumers of the information. Measures should emphasize meaningful patient outcomes rather than simply the more easily assessed processes of care, though it is of value to define and support the link between these two types of data. Special consideration should be given to measures that evaluate patient experiences and access to care. Consistent with the fundamental principle of "first, do no harm," it is vital that new measures be able to detect evidence of unintended adverse consequences as quickly as possible.

To be of maximum use, lessons learned through the measurement of performance and the subsequent analysis of performance data should be publicly reported. This information should be communicated quickly and clearly in a manner that makes it useful to a wide variety of decision makers—patients, health care providers, payers, health plans, and regulators.

AN ACTIVE LEARNING SYSTEM

Lessons learned from those pay-for-performance programs already in place (see Chapter 2) have considerable potential to enrich the practical understanding of effective design principles for such programs: those that will achieve desired change without incurring significant adverse unintended consequences. The committee envisions a learning system that will focus on the impact of pay for performance on Medicare beneficiaries, but optimally will be able to identify safeguards and benefits that could be generalized to other patient populations and to programs in the private sector. The knowledge base supporting the effectiveness of the pay-for-performance concept is currently incomplete (Petersen et al., 2006); nevertheless, considerable program assessment and guidance are possible now.

To achieve success with the greatest efficiency, actual experience with pay for performance must be accurately and objectively assessed, and the assessment results—both best practices and practices that produce adverse consequences—disseminated to those who need to make use of them. This learning system will require definition and coordination at the national level; the Medicare program is well positioned to take the lead in implementing this function. To be an effective leader, Medicare must collaborate with other public and private efforts in pay for performance. Examination of the collective experience with pay for performance and coordination of research will help advance learning and the entire research agenda. This collaboration should also lead to an alignment of pay-for-performance programs in order to reduce provider confusion and aid in achieving program goals.

The committee proposes that an active learning system be developed and incorporated into any Medicare pay-for-performance program; indeed, such a system, properly designed, will inform and guide the activities of the program itself. The active learning system should have the following characteristics and capabilities:

- Focus data collection efforts on a robust set of performance measures that address national health care goals.
- Collect, aggregate, analyze, and disseminate data in a fashion that allows for timely decision making.
- Facilitate real-time program modifications based on evidence of benefits or adverse effects.

The passage of time, coupled with objective reflection, provides both a filter and a lens for program assessment. Caution, not tentativeness or hesitation, should characterize the implementation of a pay-for-performance program. An effective learning system seeks to instill an attitude of openness and inquiry that recognizes these programs as works in progress that should be guided, validated, and enhanced by data. The system should also create a climate in which modifications based on experience are welcomed.

Learning organizations have five key elements (Senge, 1990):

- Systems thinking—looking at the dynamics of the system as a whole and in the long term, especially the interactions among individual parts of the system.
- Personal mastery—learning and vision at the individual level, including the individual's recognition of his or her role in the system.
- Mental models—examination of how individuals approach problems; in a learning organization, individuals must learn how to recognize their own perceptions and work at being open to new models.
- Building of a shared vision—creation of a picture of the future that is shared and desired by all individuals in the system, and therefore leads to increased enthusiasm and clarity.

• Team learning—a process of using and enhancing the capabilities of individuals within the system, including ongoing dialogue, to achieve the shared vision.

Effective learning organizations also have strong leaders involved in creating the guiding ideals of the system, committing to and managing the shared vision, and helping to empower the individuals in the system. It is important for the Centers for Medicare and Medicaid Services (CMS) to assume this leadership role in the initiation of a successful learning system within a pay-for-performance program in Medicare.

All of the elements of a good learning organization also depend on an ongoing dialogue among the members of the organization. Such a dialogue includes continuous examination and reflection, as practiced commonly in the rapid-cycle improvement approach espoused by Shewhart and Deming (Value Based Management.net, 2006). In this approach, a group or individual learns about the consequences of an action and then responds to those results to improve the system (commonly known as a PDCA or PDSA cycle: Plan-Do-Check/Study-Act). This cycle involves planning a small change in a process, executing the change, studying the results, and ultimately taking action to react to the results. In a pay-for-performance program, this type of cycle could be used continuously to improve the program and react immediately to any consequences detected—either to expand upon a change that produces benefits or curtail a change that produces adverse effects.

Many others have studied the important elements of learning organizations that can help achieve continuous improvement (Garvin, 1993; Senge, 1996; Ferlie and Shortell, 2001; Frankl and Gibbons-Carr, 2001; Garcarz and Chambers, 2003; Rushmer et al., 2004). In the United Kingdom, Garcarz and colleagues (2003) developed a toolkit for creating a learning organization. Box 6-1 presents a list of the factors they identified as necessary for effective learning.

While many theories and perspectives exist as to what makes a learning system successful, there are certain overlapping elements CMS should consider when designing a pay-for-performance program in Medicare: providing strong leadership; developing a shared vision; creating an environment that allows for learning from experience (including mistakes); and, especially, considering the program as a whole, including the interactions among all individual elements.

RESEARCH AGENDA

Performance Measurement

The first report in the *Pathways* series, *Performance Measurement: Accelerating Improvement* (IOM, 2006b), proposed an aggressive agenda for

BOX 6-1   Factors Necessary for Effective Learning to Take Place

Shared vision
Leadership
Empowerment of the workforce
Culture enabling learning from mistakes
Consumer focus
Commitment to teamwork
Knowledge management systems
Education, training, and development needs analysis
Appraisal, performance, and personal development plans
Identified and protected education and training budget
Opportunity to apply new skills and knowledge
Sustained change and improvement
Time for learning and reflection
Feedback and evaluation

SOURCE: Garcarz et al., 2003.

further research. As articulated in that report, to help realize the vision of quality health care articulated in the *Quality Chasm* report (IOM, 2001), three aims of care should receive particular focus in the development of new performance measures: efficiency, equity, and patient-centeredness (IOM, 2001). The *Performance Measurement* report also called for measures to better assess the quality of care offered during a patient's transition from one provider setting to another (e.g., from hospital to nursing home or from home to emergency department); such transitions have previously been identified as problematic periods during which errors are made, and important aspects of the comprehensive care plan are overlooked (Moore et al., 2003; Coleman and Berenson, 2004; Coleman and Fox, 2004; Coleman et al., 2005). Additionally, standards of care for patients with multiple chronic diseases are lacking. These patients are frequent users of the health care delivery system, seeing a variety of providers and utilizing many resources. Development of such standards is imperative to better understand how best to treat these patients who may derive most benefit from these efforts.

Numerous challenges must be faced in the development, implementation, and ongoing evaluation of performance measures that can align payment incentives with quality health care. Multiple methodological considerations—risk adjustment reflecting patient populations of varying acuity, small sample sizes at the individual practitioner level, comparative weighting of measures based on their contribution to achieving identified goals, and attribution of responsibility among multiple providers participating in the care of a single patient—have already been identified as high-priority areas for further research to better asses the true impact of payment incentives.

Development of an Evidence Base

Many conclusions in this report are based on an analysis of reasonable alternatives rather than a firmly established, rich evidence base. Much additional data about pay for performance must be gathered, aggregated, and analyzed to inform decision makers. Full advantage should be taken of the research potential of every pay-for-performance program that is implemented; in particular, the committee reiterates the importance of conducting an ongoing assessment of any program implemented within Medicare.

CMS should carry out demonstration projects to evaluate options that are theoretically sound but untested. Such projects could limit risks and accelerate progress in realignment of reimbursement by confirming benefits and averting undue hardships for beneficiaries or providers. The following are examples of questions that should be addressed by demonstration projects or by other methods:

- What is the threshold magnitude for rewards that will lead to significant changes in provider behavior? Does it vary among different types of providers (such as hospitals versus physicians)?
- What are the effects of rewarding incremental change by recognizing relative improvement in practice versus rewarding only attainment of an absolute level of performance?
- What criteria should be used to determine how rewards should be structured? Does the selected structure equitably recognize shared accountability among providers?
- Should performance measures that enhance value to the patient always be the first priority for rewards? To what extent is control of costs advantageous to patients?
- Should performance measures that recognize achievement in different domains of performance—clinical quality, patient-centeredness, and efficiency—be weighted differently in determining rewards?
- How can a pay-for-performance program promote comprehensive rather than episodic care?
- Should rewards be made at the organizational level or at the level of the individual provider?
- Are virtual groups a feasible alternative?
- How can best practices be identified and incorporated into a pay-for-performance program?

- Is risk adjustment necessary to balance effectiveness and fairness?
- How can a pay-for-performance program promote efficient health care without compromising clinical quality or patient-centeredness?
- How should a pay-for-performance program be structured to sustain meaningful quality improvement over time?

A detailed analysis of methods for answering these research questions is beyond the scope of this report; however, a broad range of methodologies should be considered. In particular, mining of large databases offers real potential, particularly if the public and private sectors can be linked in a meaningful way.

Oversight

It appears likely that oversight of any significant program of research and evaluation for pay-for-performance initiatives will have to occur at the national level, both within and outside the Medicare program and consistent with national consensus goals for health care. The National Quality Coordination Board proposed in the first report in the *Pathways* series (IOM, 2006b) is a particularly applicable model for this purpose. The Board might make use of the services of other organizations, both public (CMS, the Agency for Healthcare Research and Quality, the Government Accountability Office) and private (the Joint Commission on Accreditation of Healthcare Organizations, the National Committee for Quality Assurance, the National Quality Forum), that are already performing some of these functions with demonstrated ability.

SUMMARY

This chapter has addressed issues related to the future directions for monitoring and evaluation of a pay-for-performance program within Medicare and proposed a research agenda. Key points made are as follows:

- Monitoring, evaluation, and research will depend upon the development of valid and robust measures, as well as a real-time monitoring system.
- A successful pay-for-performance program must encompass the elements of a true learning system, including having strong leadership, a shared vision, and an environment that allows for action in response to observations (including the opportunity to learn from mistakes).
- A research agenda must address the fundamentals of performance measurement as necessary to align payment incentives with quality improvement. In the short term, the development of new measures should address

in particular the domains of clinical quality, patient-centeredness, and efficiency, and should also be focused on enhanced care coordination. Research should attempt as well to build an evidence base upon which the design of future pay-for-performance programs can be based.

REFERENCES

Coleman EA, Berenson RA. 2004. Lost in transition: Challenges and opportunities for improving the quality of transitional care. *Annals of Internal Medicine* 141(7):533–536.

Coleman EA, Fox PD. 2004. One patient, many places: Managing health care transitions, Part III: Financial incentives and getting started. *Annals of Long-Term Care* 12(11): 14–16.

Coleman EA, Mahoney E, Parry C. 2005. Assessing the quality of preparation for posthospital care from the patient's perspective: The care transitions measure. *Medical Care* 43(3):246–255.

Ferlie EB, Shortell SM. 2001. Improving the quality of health care in the United Kingdom and the United States: A framework for change. *The Milbank Quarterly* 79(2):281–315.

Frankl SN, Gibbons-Carr M. 2001. Creating a school without walls and building a learning organization: A case study. *Journal of Dental Education* 65(11):1253–1263; discussion 1264.

Garcarz W, Chambers R. 2003. Creating and sustaining a learning organisation in the NHS. *Quality in Primary Care* 11(4):255–256.

Garcarz W, Fisher A, Chambers R, Ellis S. 2003. *Towards a Learning Organization Toolkit.* Commissioned by the Shropshire and Staffordshire Workforce Development Confederation. Unpublished.

Garvin D. 1993. Building a learning organization. *Harvard Business Review* 71(4):78–91.

IOM (Institute of Medicine). 2001. *Crossing the Quality Chasm: A New Health System for the 21st Century.* Washington, DC: National Academy Press.

IOM. 2006a. *Medicare's Quality Improvement Organization Program: Maximizing Potential.* Washington, DC: The National Academies Press.

IOM. 2006b. *Performance Measurement: Accelerating Improvement.* Washington, DC: The National Academies Press.

Moore C, Wisnivesky J, Williams S, McGinn T. 2003. Medical errors related to discontinuity of care from an inpatient to an outpatient setting. *Journal of General Internal Medicine* 18(8):646–651.

Petersen L, Woodard L, Urech T, Daw C, Sookanan S. 2006. Does pay-for-performance improve the quality of health care? *Annals of Internal Medicine* 145(4):265–272.

Rushmer R, Kelly D, Lough M, Wilkinson JE, Davies HTO. 2004. Introducing the learning practice—I. The characteristics of learning organizations in primary care. *Journal of Evaluation in Clinical Practice* 10(3):375–386.

Senge P. 1990. *The Fifth Discipline: The Art and Practice of the Learning Organization.* New York: Doubleday.

Senge P. 1996. Building learning organizations. *MIT Sloan Management Review* 24(1): 96–104.

Value Based Management.net. 2006. *The Deming Cycle.* [Online]. Available: http://www.valuebasedmanagement.net/methods_demingcycle.html [accessed May 25, 2006].

Appendixes

A

Selected Medicare Prospective Payment Systems

ACUTE CARE HOSPITALS, INPATIENT

The inpatient hospital prospective payment system (PPS), which was established in 1983, uses a preset payment schedule based on a patient's principal diagnosis at discharge, comorbidities, and complications. The service unit is a patient stay. The fixed payment amounts are intended to cover the average costs of all services, supplies, and elements of care an efficient hospital would need to treat the average patient in a specified diagnosis-related group (DRG). There are 524 distinct DRGs, each of which encompasses "patients with similar clinical problems that are expected to require similar amounts of hospital resources" (MedPAC, 2005a). Some cases will cost the hospital more and others less than actual Medicare payments for a particular diagnosis. While these "bundled" payments are indexed to account for geographic differences in labor and other input costs, all hospitals within an area receive the same base payments for DRGs regardless of quality (Worzala et al., 2003). Hospital-specific adjustments that take the form of a percentage increase in all payments are made for institutions serving a disproportionate share of low-income and uninsured patients and teaching hospitals.

The acute inpatient hospital PPS provides an incentive to manage the costs of inputs needed for care. Hospitals can manage their costs by eliminating unnecessary services, reducing the intensity of services per case, bargaining hard over input prices, shortening lengths of stay, increasing the volume of less complex cases within any particular DRG, and reducing the volume of cases in DRGs for which Medicare's preset payment does not cover the costs of the average case. The impact of the hospital inpatient PPS on the quality of hospital care is unclear. Early concerns that the DRG payment system would lead to stinting on care and an inappropriate shortening of hospital stays appear largely to have been unfounded. MedPAC's most recent assessment of trends found lower in-hospital and 30-day mortality rates, improvement in measures of appropriateness of care and clinical effectiveness, and some increases and some decreases in measures of adverse events (MedPAC, 2006).

ACUTE CARE HOSPITALS, OUTPATIENT

The implementation of inpatient PPS promoted a shift of care to outpatient departments because hospitals continued to be reimbursed for such care on a retrospective, cost basis. To reduce this incentive, a hospital outpatient PPS was introduced in 2000. Like the inpatient PPS, the outpatient system groups services that are similar clinically and costwise into one of about 850 ambulatory payment classification (APC) categories, each with its own payment rate. Additional APCs are designated for new technologies—those for which the Centers for Medicare and Medicaid Services has insufficient data—which are grouped together by cost, not clinical similarity. There are also pass-through payments that cover the costs of particular new drugs; costs of biologicals and devices used in the delivery of services; outlier payments for cases that are unusually expensive relative to the preset payment rate; and adjustments for rural, low-volume facilities.

Compared with the inpatient PPS, the outpatient system provides somewhat weaker incentives for efficiencies because the APC service bundles are not as broad as those of the DRGs, and the use of certain new technologies is encouraged. The volume of outpatient services continues to grow rapidly as procedures once requiring a hospital stay can now be performed safely on an outpatient basis. There is little systematic knowledge about trends in the quality of outpatient care or the impact that the outpatient PPS may have had on the quality of care.

SKILLED NURSING FACILITIES

Skilled nursing facilities (SNFs) shifted from cost-based reimbursement to a PPS in 1998. Under the PPS, SNFs are paid set per diem rates for each patient. Based on periodic assessments, patients with similar needs and characteristics are placed in one of 53 resource utilization groups, each with its own payment rate. These rates, which are the sum of a nursing component, a therapy component, and a routine services component, are intended to cover all routine care and ancillary services. Additional payments are made for certain rare but high-cost ancillary services, such as an outpatient hospital scan. The per diem base payments are adjusted for geographic differences in labor costs. Nontherapy ancillary services, such as tracheostomy and ventilator care, and certain prescription drugs, while included in the nursing component of the base rate, were not included in the case mix indexes, so the base payments do not appropriately reflect the resource needs of certain extensive care patients (MedPAC, 2006). Recently, payments for patients needing extensive (nontherapy) services were reduced absolutely and in comparison with those for patients needing therapies, and that change may explain the relatively longer delays such patients encounter in accessing SNF care (MedPAC, 2005b). Information is insufficient for making judgments about the quality of care provided in individual facilities or industrywide; only three measures collected through the patient assessment and reporting system known as the nursing home Minimum Data Set relate to the quality of SNF care.

HOME HEALTH

Medicare's market share nationally for free-standing home health care was 32 percent in 2003; the percent for hospital-based home health care was not available (MedPAC, 2006). Until the mid-1990s, home health agencies received cost-based reimbursement from Medicare. The number of Medicare patients, the number of services provided per case, and the number of agencies grew quickly in the early 1990s. Although the number of visits for each case had to be approved by the Medicare fiscal intermediary, the cost-based system encouraged agencies to provide as many visits as would be allowed. In 1998 Medicare implemented a 2-year interim payment system to provide a transition to prospective payment. The interim system included a financial incentive to cut the number of visits per case when possible. The number of participating agencies dropped by approximately 30 percent from 1997 to 2000, indicating the impact of Medicare's payment policy, along with strong new regulatory efforts to control fraud and abuse in the home health industry.

Under the home health PPS, implemented in 2000, the unit of payment is an episode, which includes all services needed during a 60-day period. If the patient needs care for a longer period, the home health agency receives another episode payment. The episode includes skilled nursing care; physical, occupational, and speech therapy; and medical social work and aide services. Patients are assigned to one of 80 Home Health Resource Groups based on their functional status, clinical condition, and likely use of various services. Outlier payments are made for particularly costly episodes, and reduced payments are made for episodes that require fewer than five visits, for transfer cases, and for patients that have a significant change in status during an episode.

Lacking a sophisticated case mix adjustment that accurately reflects the likely resource needs of the patient, providers have an incentive to decrease the number of visits per episode and to increase the number of episodes per patient. The impact of the payment system can be seen during the transition period, between 1997 and 2002: the average visits per episode dropped from 36 to 19 and the average length of stay from 106 to 56 days (MedPAC, 2005d).

Performance measures of home health services show quality has improved slightly or remained stable over the last couple of years, but that trend cannot be related to specific changes in payment. What confounds judgments about the impact of payment incentives on the use of home health services and their quality is the lack of specific methods and guidelines for identifying patients in need of such services, what specific services they need, and whether home health is the most appropriate source for that care. This situation is not unique to home health care; it is typical of all post–acute care settings in which patients can receive similar services from different types of providers that receive different amounts and types of payments.

OUTPATIENT DIALYSIS SERVICES

The payment for outpatient dialysis services has two parts: the slightly larger part is a prospective composite payment that covers the bundle of services associated with a dialysis treatment, and the smaller part covers certain separately billable drugs and supplements, such as erythropoietin, vitamin D, and iron. Dialysis facilities also receive payments for laboratory tests not included in the composite rate. The composite payment is adjusted for the patient's age, body mass, and body surface area and for geographic differences in wages and other costs. While the base payment is the same for hemodialysis and peritoneal dialysis and for in-center or home dialysis, hospital-based facilities receive $4 more per treatment.

The payment system had created incentives for providers to increase the efficiency of the composite-covered services and to increase use of the separately covered drugs and supplements because the latter payment had been based on the average wholesale price of the products, which exceeded the centers' acquisition costs. The Medicare Prescription Drug, Improvement, and Modernization Act of 2003 (Public Law 108-173) required that beginning in 2006, the drug payment be the average sales price plus 6 percent, and that the savings be added to the composite rate. This less generous drug payment was intended to slow the growth in drug spending without jeopardizing the quality of care for dialysis patients. While the volume of services has been growing, the proportion of people receiving services at home has been shrinking (MedPAC, 2006). Because the payments are location neutral, the latter trend may indicate a perception on the part of providers that home dialysis is more costly to provide or that patients find it less desirable. The dialysis program has its own quality improvement organizations that have documented improvements in care between 1999 and 2003, but it is too soon to tell whether recent changes in the payment system have had any effect on this trend.

PHYSICIANS

Medicare pays for services provided by physicians and other medical professionals who can charge directly—such as dentists, optometrists, podiatrists, chiropractors, psychologists, clinical social workers, nurse midwives, certified registered nurse anesthetists, physician assistants, nurse practitioners, clinical nurse specialists, physical therapists, occupational therapists, and registered dietitians—under the physician fee schedule. This schedule assigns a payment amount to each of more than 7,000 procedures, visit types, and other diagnostic and therapeutic services. The scope of some of the services—such as a flu shot—is quite narrow, while that of others—such as the office and hospital visits and surgery associated with a hip replacement—is quite broad. Over 74 percent of public and private payers, including state Medicaid programs, have adopted components of the Medicare system for reimbursing physicians (AAP, 2005).

The specific amount of the payment is based on the relative costliness of the professional work, practice expenses, and liability insurance needed to provide the service. The latter two components are adjusted for geographic differences in costs. Because the initial methodology for determining the relative value of the professional work involved in providing specific services was based on calculations of the resources used in care, the time involved, the complexity of procedures, and physician training,[1] the fee schedule tends to reward specialty care at higher rates relative to primary care.

The annual updates to the physician fee schedule are governed by the sustainable growth rate, which, broadly speaking, limits the growth in per beneficiary physician fee schedule expenditures to the growth in per capita gross domestic product. Recent rapid growth in the volume and intensity of services and congressional interventions to stave off payment reductions have created a situation in which the updates for the physician fee schedule are projected to be negative for at least the next 7 years.

---

[1]These costs are divided into three components: the amount of physician work that goes into a service, the practice expense for the provision of the service, and the professional liability expense for the provision of the service. The relative value is also multiplied by Geographic Practice Cost Indices for each Medicare locality, and then translated into a dollar amount by an annually adjusted conversion factor.

Since the system is based on paying per service provided, it tends to penalize rather than reward physicians who use fewer resources or services to achieve a given level of quality or outcome (Wilensky, 2005). But the physician or other provider will receive additional payment if the service resulted in a complication and had to be repeated or followed by corrective procedures. The payment system also tends to offer higher rates for new technologies while providing few incentives to use older, lower-cost technologies that may be equally effective.

MEDICARE ADVANTAGE

Medicare Advantage (MA) plans are paid a capitated amount for each participant each month, the size of which depends on the plan's bid, a benchmark, and the risk characteristics of the beneficiary. For local plans, those that offer their services on a county-by-county basis, the benchmark is the county MA payment rate that existed before 2006, updated each year by the increase in national per beneficiary fee-for-service (FFS) spending. The old payment rates generally exceeded the average per capita expenditures for FFS, in some counties by a considerable amount. Some MA plans benefited from minimum payment floors or blended local–national rates that were intended to attract MA plans into areas with low FFS spending; others were boosted by a guaranteed minimum update; and still others were advantaged by inconsistencies in the methodology used to set the rate. For regional plans, the preferred provider organizations that offer service throughout one of the 26 state or multistate regions, the benchmark is a weighted average of the local benchmarks.

Each year, Medicare compares plan bids with the relevant benchmark for providing the comprehensive bundle of services mandated by Medicare Parts A and B (except hospice services) for an average beneficiary. If the bid is below the benchmark, the plan is paid its bid plus three-fourths of the difference between the benchmark and the bid. The plan must use the "excess" payment for additional (nonrequired) benefits, reduced cost sharing, or Part B or Part D premium reductions. Plans bidding above the benchmark are paid the benchmark and must charge their participants the difference between their bid and the benchmark. The basic payment is adjusted for an enrollee's risk profile using a methodology that incorporates information on the individual's demographic characteristics and previous use of hospital inpatient and ambulatory services. The quality of care in MA plans is measured more fully and there is a longer history of performance data collection than is the case for FFS Medicare. The Health Plan Employer Data and Information Set is used for data collection, and those measures show general improvement over time; some measures remain low, however, and there is substantial variation among overall plan scores (MedPAC,

2005c). It is unclear how the payment methods have affected quality and, given the major changes in those methods over the last decade, it would be difficult to attribute quality change to any specific incentive in the payment system.

REFERENCES

AAP (American Academy of Pediatrics). 2005. *2006 RBRVS: What Is It and How Does It Affect Pediatrics?* [Online]. Available: http://www.aap.org/visit/rbrvsbrochure.pdf [accessed December 7, 2005].

MedPAC (Medicare Payment Advisory Commission). 2005a. *Hospital Acute Inpatient Services Payment System.* Washington, DC: MedPAC.

MedPAC. 2005b. *Report to the Congress: Medicare Payment Policy.* Washington, DC: MedPAC.

MedPAC. 2005c. *A Data Book: Healthcare Spending and the Medicare Program.* Washington, DC: MedPAC.

MedPAC. 2005d. *MedPAC Data Runs.* Washington, DC: MedPAC.

MedPAC. 2006. *Report to the Congress: Medicare Payment Policy.* Washington, DC: MedPAC.

Wilensky GR. 2005. The twin policy challenges of Medicare physician payment and Medicaid. *Health Affairs* w5-333–w5-334.

Worzala C, Pettengill J, Ashby J. 2003. Challenges and opportunities for Medicare's original prospective payment system. *Health Affairs* 22(6):175–182.

B

Review of the Evidence

TABLE B-1   Articles Identified as Assessing Explicit Financial Incentives and
Health Care Quality from a Systematic Review of the Literature After
Applying Study Inclusion and Exclusion Criteria[a]

Reference	Study Design	Incentives
Norton, 1992	RCT (2 arms); November 1980 to April 1983; 36 SNFs (18 study facilities; 18 control facilities)	Level: payment system Type: bonus Duration: admission incentive up to 4 y; outcome and discharge incentives 1 to 2 y Admission incentive: per diem bonus for type D ($5) and E ($3 to $28) patients (vs. $36 reimbursement) Outcome incentive: improved health status within 90 d (measured by ADL classification); $126 to $370 per case (range of bonus) Discharge incentive: timely discharge and resident did not return within 90 d; $60 to $230 (range of bonus); type A patients not eligible Payment frequency: NS
Shen, 2003	CBA; FY 1991 to 1995; 5552 clients (2367 OSA clients; 3185 Medicaid clients)	Level: payment system Type: PBC Duration: FY 1993 to 1995 Description: additional funds based on efficiency, effectiveness, and service to special populations Efficiency: minimum service delivery (% of contracted amount); minimum service to primary clients (% of units delivered) Effectiveness: abstinence/drug-free 30 d before termination; reduction of use of primary substance abuse problem; maintaining employment; employability; employment improvement; reduction in number of problems with employer; reduction in absenteeism; not arrested; participation in self-help during treatment; reduction of problems with spouse/family members Special populations: female; age 0 to 19 y; age ≥50 y; corrections; homeless; concurrent psychological problems; history of IV drug use; polydrug use Payment frequency: yearly

Domains of Quality	Analysis and Results	Overall Effect[b]	Methodologic Strength[c]
Access; outcome	Markov model Experimental homes admitted more type D and E patients (sicker patients) than control homes Patients in experimental homes were more likely to be discharged to home or to an ICF and had less likelihood of hospital admission or death ($P < 0.001$)	Positive	3
Access	Probit specification (regression) Significant decrease in the likelihood that an OSA patient was a "most severe user" after PBC implementation compared with the likelihood of a Medicaid (control) patient; coefficient = −0.74; t-value = 3.26; $P \leq 0.01$	Negative	2

continues

TABLE B-1 Continued

Reference	Study Design	Incentives
Clark et al., 1995	CBA; July 1992; 7 CMHCs; 185 clients (95 in TCM and 90 in CTT)	Level: provider group Type: enhanced FFS Duration: NA Description: CMHCs received $15.75 per 15 min spent in community settings delivering MIMS Payment frequency: FFS
Hillman et al., 1998	RCT (2 arms); 1993 to 1995; 52 PC sites (26 intervention; 26 control)	Level: provider group Type: bonus Duration: 18 mo Description: compliance with cancer screening for women age ≥ 50 y; aggregate compliance scores and improvement in scores over time; full and partial bonuses (20%; 10% of capitation); range of bonus per site, $570 to $1260 Payment frequency: every 6 mo
Kouides et al., 1998	RCT (2 arms); September to December 1991; 54 solo/group practices (27 intervention; 27 control)	Level: provider group Type: bonus Duration: 4 mo Description: influenza immunization rate ($8 standard fee); if rate >70%, bonus of $0.80 per immunization; if rate >85%, bonus of $1.60 Payment frequency: one time (end of study)

Domains of Quality	Analysis and Results	Overall Effect[b]	Methodologic Strength[c]
Access	Student *t*-test for paired comparisons; MANOVA Student *t*-test: average weekly time spent in community treatment per client increased after the payment change (30.71 min vs. 38.61 min; $P < 0.05$) Office-based case management weekly time per client decreased (32.96 min vs. 23.31 min; $P < 0.001$) Total case manager average weekly time per client was not significantly different (63.68 min vs. 61.93 min) MANOVA: after the payment change, center-based treatment time decreased (F-value = 10.41; $P = 0.001$). The increase in community minutes had an F-value of 3.72 ($P = 0.055$). Program type and Medicaid status were not associated with change in time in community vs. mental health center	Partial effect	2
Process	Repeated-measures ANOVA Absolute increase in total mean compliance scores for intervention group from baseline was 26.3%; control group was 26.4%. No significant differences between the groups	No effect	3
Process	Linear regression Absolute increase in immunization rates (from 1990 [baseline] to 1991) was 6.8%; $P = 0.03$	Positive	3

continues

TABLE B-1 Continued

Reference	Study Design	Incentives
Hillman et al., 1999	RCT (3 arms); 1993 to 1995; 49 PC sites (19 FB+I; 15 FBO; 15 control)	Level: provider group Type: bonus Duration: 18 mo Description: pediatric immunizations; well-child visits; bonuses based on total compliance score for quality indicators; full and partial bonuses (20%; 10% of site's total 6-mo capitation for pediatric members ≤age 6 y); 3 highest-scoring sites received full bonus; next 3 received partial bonus; most improved sites received partial bonus; average bonus, $2,000 (range, $772 to $4682) Payment frequency: every 6 mo
Christensen et al., 2000	RCT (2 arms); February 1994 to September 1995; 200 pharmacies (110 intervention; 90 control)	Level: provider group Type: enhanced FFS Duration: 20 mo Description: $4 for cognitive services interventions (< 6 min); $6 for ≥ 6 min; cognitive services are judgmental or educational services provided by the pharmacist to the patient, such as consulting the prescriber about a suboptimal dose Payment frequency: FFS
Casalino et al., 2003	Cross-sectional survey; September 2000 to September 2001; 1040 physician organizations (no patient-level data included)	Level: provider group Type: better contracts with health plans; bonuses Duration: not ascertained in survey Description: not ascertained in survey Payment frequency: not ascertained in survey

Domains of Quality	Analysis and Results	Overall Effect[b]	Methodologic Strength[c]
Process	Repeated-measures ANOVA Absolute increase in total mean compliance scores from baseline: FB+I, 17.2%; FBO, 22.6%; control, 22.6% Differences in compliance score improvement between groups: FB+I vs. control, 5.9%; FBO vs. control, 11.3% No significant differences between the groups	No effect	3
Process	Student t-test Mean rate, 1.59 interventions per 100 Medicaid prescriptions (study pharmacies) vs. 0.67 (controls); $P < 0.001$	Positive	2
Process	Multivariate linear regression Receiving better contracts for quality was associated with an increase of 0.74 CMP implemented ($P = 0.007$). Receiving a bonus for scoring well on quality measures was not associated with CMP implementation ($P = 0.08$)	Partial effect	1

continues

TABLE B-1 Continued

Reference	Study Design	Incentives
McMenamin et al., 2003	Cross-sectional survey; September 2000 to September 2001; 1104 physician organizations	Level: provider group Type: financial incentives; additional income; better contracts with health plans Duration: not ascertained in survey Description: not ascertained in survey Payment frequency: not ascertained in survey
Roski et al., 2003	RCT (3 arms); May 1999 to June 2000; 37 PC sites (13 incentive; 9 incentive + registry; 15 control)	Level: provider group Type: bonus Duration: 12 mo Description: 75% of patients with smoking status identified/documented at the last visit; 65% of patients with quitting advice documented at the last visit (targets set at approximately 15% above the average from 2 y before study); bonuses, $5000 for sites with 1–7 providers and $10,000 for sites with ≥8 providers Outcome measured: 7-d sustained abstinence from smoking (not associated with financial incentive) Payment frequency: one time (end of study)

Domains of Quality	Analysis and Results	Overall Effect[b]	Method-ologic Strength[c]
Process	Multivariate logistic regression Receiving financial incentives from HMOs increased the adjusted odds of having a smoking cessation intervention for 6 of the 7 organizational supports (OR, 2.13 to 14.46; $P < 0.038$) Receiving additional income from health plans for performance on quality measures: 2 of 7 organizational supports (OR, 1.49, 1.90; $P < 0.033$) Receiving better contracts with health plans was not associated with supporting smoking cessation interventions Examples of organizational supports include offering smoking cessation health promotion programs and giving providers nicotine replacement starter kits to distribute to patients	Partial effect	1
Process	Logistic regression, clustering at the practice level Change in tobacco use status identification: incentive group had increased 14.1%; incentive + registry group increased 8.1%; control group increased 6.2%; $P = 0.009$ Change in providing quitting advice to patients: incentive group increased 24.2%; incentive + registry increased 18.3%; control increased 18.3%. No significant difference across the study groups The quitting rate (7-d sustained abstinence) was 22.4% for the incentive group; 21.7% for the incentive + registry group; 19.2% for the control group. No significant difference across the study groups	Partial effect	2

continues

TABLE B-1   Continued

Reference	Study Design	Incentives
Rosenthal et al., 2005	CBA; October 2001 to April 2004; 163 provider groups contracted with PacifiCare Health Systems in California (provider groups in the Pacific Northwest were the comparison group)	Level: provider group Type: bonus Duration: July 2003 to April 2004 (10 mo) Description: incentive payout based on provider's groups ability to reach or exceed target rates for cervical cancer screening, mammography, and hemoglobin A_{1c} testing for diabetic patients Incentive reward: $0.23 PMPM Payment frequency: quarterly
Grady et al., 1997	RCT (3 arms); 1 year (NS); 61 community-based primary care practices (20 cue and reward; 18 cue; 23 control [total of 95 physicians]); cues were posters in waiting rooms and chart reminder stickers	Level: physician Type: bonus ($50 for a 50% referral rate) Duration: 6 mo Description: "token" reward, based on the percentage referred for mammography during quarterly audit Payment frequency: 1 per quarterly audit; rewards given last 2 quarters
Fairbrother et al., 1999	RCT (4 arms); July 1995 to July 1996; 60 physicians (15 bonus; 15 enhanced FFS; 15 feedback only; 15 control)	Level: physician Type: bonus and FFS Duration: 12 mo Description: patients' up-to-date coverage for pediatric immunizations Bonuses: $1000 (20% improvement from baseline); $2500 (40% improvement); $5000 (80% up-to-date) Enhanced FFS: $5 per vaccine given within 30 d of its coming due; $15 for each visit at which >1 vaccine was due and all were given Payment frequency: every 4 mo
Safran et al., 2000	Cross-sectional survey; January to April, October 1996; physicians in 8 IPA/network HMOs (2761 patients)	Level: physician Type: not ascertained in survey Duration: not ascertained in survey Description: survey of health plan executives elicited information about use of financial incentives regarding patient satisfaction Payment frequency: not ascertained in survey

Domains of Quality	Analysis and Results	Overall Effect[b]	Methodologic Strength[c]
Process	Differences-in-differences analysis using generalized estimating equations Improvement in cervical cancer screening rates before and after the quality incentive program was statistically significant between the intervention and comparison groups (difference, 3.6%; $P = 0.02$). Improvements in mammography screening rates and hemoglobin A_{1c} testing were not statistically significant	Partial effect	2
Process	Repeated-measures ANOVA The financial incentive arm was not significantly different from the control arm	No effect	2
Process	Linear and logistic regression Bonus group improved significantly in documented up-to-date immunization status, with an overall change of 25.3% ($P < 0.01$), but none of the other groups improved significantly compared with controls	Partial effect	3
Patient experience	Linear regression Financial incentives concerning patient satisfaction were related to increase in score on primary care scale completed by patients on 2 of the 4 aspects of primary care assessed (access, physicians' knowledge of patients, clinician–patient communication, and interpersonal treatment) Access to care ($\beta = 2.57$; $P < 0.01$) and dimensions of comprehensiveness of care ($\beta = 2.00$ for knowledge of patient; $P < 0.05$) and preventive counseling ($\beta = 3.50$; $P < 0.05$)	Partial effect	1

continues

TABLE B-1 Continued

Reference	Study Design	Incentives
Fairbrother et al., 2001	RCT (3 arms); July 1997 to July 1998; 57 physicians (24 bonus; 12 FFS; 21 control)	Level: physician Type: bonus and FFS Duration: 16 mo Description: patients' up-to-date coverage for pediatric immunizations Bonuses: $1000 (30% improvement from baseline); $2500 (45% improvement); $5000 (80% up-to-date); $7500 (90% up-to-date) Enhanced FFS: $5 per vaccine given within 30 d of its coming due; $15 for each visit at which >1 vaccine was due and all were given Payment frequency: every 4 mo
Beaulieu and Horrigan, 2005	CBA; April 2001 to January 2002; 21 PCPs contracted with Independent Health in upstate New York (476 diabetic patients); 600 Independent Health diabetic patients were the comparison group	Level: physician Type: bonus Duration: 8 mo Description: meeting target CS of ≥6.23; CS of ≥6.86; or overall 50% improvement in composite score. CS based on PCP's performance of process and outcome measures for diabetes care (e.g., LDL test, dilated retinal examination, LDL cholesterol level <2.59 mmol/L (<100 mg/dL)) Incentive rewards: CS >6.86, $3.00 PMPM (Medicare), $0.75 PMPM (commercial); CS >6.23, $1.50 PMPM (Medicare), $0.37 PMPM (commercial); 50% improvement and CS <6.23, $0.75 PMPM (Medicare), $0.18 PMPM (commercial) Payment frequency: at the conclusion of the study

Domains of Quality	Analysis and Results	Overall Effect[b]	Methodologic Strength[c]
Process	Linear and logistic regression Both the bonus and the enhanced FFS groups improved significantly in documented up-to-date immunization status, with an overall change of 5.9% ($P < 0.05$) and 7.4% ($P < 0.01$), respectively, compared with the control group	Positive	3
Process; intermediate outcome	Before and after comparison, specific test not described Patients treated by physicians in the demonstration project had statistically significant improvement (final – baseline performance) on the following process and outcomes measures ($P < 0.001$ unless otherwise noted): second hemoglobin A_1c test (25.5% difference); LDL cholesterol test (18.3% difference); diabetic retinal examination (25.6% difference); nephropathy test (37.0% difference); foot examination (45.4% difference); hemoglobin A_1c level <9.5% (13.9% difference); LDL cholesterol level <2.59 mmol/L (<100 mg/dL) (10.5% difference); LDL cholesterol level <3.37 mmol/L (< 130 mg/dL) (23.5% difference); BP < 130/80 mm Hg (6.3% difference; $P < 0.05$). No significant improvement on performing 1 hemoglobin A_1c test	Partial effect	1

continues

TABLE B-1   Continued

Reference	Study Design	Incentives
Pourat et al., 2005	Cross-sectional survey; January to May 2002; PCPs contracted with Medicaid HMOs in 8 California counties with the highest rates of *Chlamydia trachomatis* infection and Medicaid HMO enrollment	Level: physician Type: better contracts with health plans Duration: not ascertained in survey Description: HMO contracts included reimbursements for quality of care dimensions, including patient satisfaction or peer review Payment frequency: not ascertained in survey

[a]Study inclusion criteria were that the article must be an original report providing empirical results and the study must assess the relationship between an explicit financial incentive and a quantitative measure of health care quality. Articles were excluded if there was no concurrent comparison group, or if there was no baseline, pre-intervention analysis of the groups on the quality measure. ADL = activities of daily living; ANOVA = analysis of variance; BP= blood pressure; CBA = controlled before and after; CMHC = community mental health center; CMP = care management process; CS= composite score; CTT = continuous treatment team; FB+I = feedback and incentive; FBO = feedback only; FFS = fee for service; FY = fiscal year; HMO = health maintenance organization; ICF = intermediate care facility; IPA = independent practice association; IV= intravenous; LDL = low-density lipoprotein; MANOVA = multivariate analysis of variance; MIMS = mental illness management services; NA= not applicable; NS= not specified; OR = odds ratio; OSA = Office of Substance Abuse; PBC = performance-based contracting; PC = primary care; PCP = primary care physicians; PMPM = per member per month; RCT = randomized, controlled trial; SNF = skilled nursing facility; TCM = traditional case managers.

[b]Positive studies were those for which all measures of quality demonstrated a statistically significant improvement with the financial incentive. Partial effect studies showed improved performance on some measures of quality but not others. Negative studies were those for which all measures of quality demonstrated a statistically significant decrease with the financial incentive.

[c]Graded on a scale of 1 (poor) to 4 (excellent).

SOURCE: Petersen LA, Woodard LD, Urech T, Daw C, Sookanan S. 2006. Does pay-for-performance improve the quality of health care? *Annals of Internal Medicine* 145(4): 265–272.

Domains of Quality	Analysis and Results	Overall Effect[b]	Methodologic Strength[c]
Process	Chi-square, logistic regression Primary care physicians reimbursed under salary and quality of care more often adhered to annual screening of sexually active females age 15 to 19 y, compared with physicians compensated by capitation and financial performance, salary and productivity, salary and financial performance, or FFS ($P < 0.05$) The physicians with salary and quality of care incentive also more often consistently screened women age 20 to 25 y for *Chlamydia trachomatis* infection annually compared with physicians reimbursed using other payment mechanisms ($P < 0.05$)	Positive	1

REFERENCES

Beaulieu ND, Horrigan DR. 2005. Putting smart money to work for quality improvement. *Health Services Research* 40:1318–1334.

Casalino L, Gillies RR, Shortell SM, Schmittdiel JA, Bodenheimer T, Robinson JC, et al. 2003. External incentives, information technology, and organized processes to improve health care quality for patients with chronic diseases. *Journal of the American Medical Association* 289:434–441.

Christensen DB, Neil N, Fassett WE, Smith DH, Holmes G, Stergachis A. 2000. Frequency and characteristics of cognitive services provided in response to a financial incentive. *Journal of the American Pharmaceutical Association* 40:609–617.

Clark RE, Drake RE, McHugo GJ, Ackerson TH. 1995. Incentives for community treatment: Mental illness management services. *Medical Care* 33:729–738.

Fairbrother G, Hanson KL, Friedman S, Butts GC. 1999. The impact of physician bonuses, enhanced fees, and feedback on childhood immunization coverage rates. *American Journal of Public Health* 89:171–175.

Fairbrother G, Siegel MJ, Friedman S, Kory PD, Butts GC. 2001. Impact of financial incentives on documented immunization rates in the inner city: Results of a randomized controlled trial. *Ambulatory Pediatrics* 1:206–212.

Grady KE, Lemkau JP, Lee NR, Caddell C. 1997. Enhancing mammography referral in primary care. *American Journal of Preventive Medicine* 26:791–800.

Hillman AL, Ripley K, Goldfarb N, Nuamah I, Weiner J, Lusk E. 1998. Physician financial incentives and feedback: Failure to increase cancer screening in Medicaid managed care. *American Journal of Public Health* 88:1699–1701.

Hillman AL, Ripley K, Goldfarb N, Weiner J, Nuamah I, Lusk E. 1999. The use of physician financial incentives and feedback to improve pediatric preventive care in Medicaid managed care. *Pediatrics* 104:931–995.

Kouides RW, Bennett NM, Lewis B, Cappuccio JD, Barker WH, LaForce FM. 1998. Performance-based physician reimbursement and influenza immunization rates in the elderly. *American Journal of Preventive Medicine* 14:89–95.

McMenamin SB, Schauffler HH, Shortell SM, Rundall TG, Gillies RR. 2003. Support for smoking cessation interventions in physician organizations: Results from a national study. *Medical Care* 41:1396–1406.

Norton EC. 1992. Incentive regulation of nursing homes. *Journal of Health Economics* 11:105–128.

Pourat N, Rice T, Tai-Seale M, Bolan G, Nihalani J. 2005. Association between physician compensation methods and delivery of guideline-concordant STD care: Is there a link? *American Journal of Managed Care* 11:426–432.

Rosenthal MB, Frank RG, Li Z, Epstein AM. 2005. Early experience with pay-for-performance: From concept to practice. *Journal of the American Medical Association* 294:1788–1793.

Roski J, Jeddeloh R, An L, Lando H, Hannan P, Hall C, et al. 2003. The impact of financial incentives and a patient registry on preventive care quality: Increasing provider adherence to evidence-based smoking cessation practice guidelines. *American Journal of Preventive Medicine* 36:291–299.

Safran DG, Rogers WH, Tarlov AR, Inui T, Taira DA, Montgomery JE, et al. 2000. Organizational and financial characteristics of health plans: Are they related to primary care performance? *Archives of Internal Medicine* 160:69–76.

Shen Y. 2003. Selection incentives in a performance-based contracting system. *Health Services Research* 38:535–552.

C

Comparison of Various Professional Groups' Pay-for-Performance Position Statements

TABLE C-1 Comparison Among Nonspecialist Groups' Pay-for-Performance Position Statements

Design Issue	American Medical Association	American College of Physicians	American Academy of Family Physicians
Participation (Voluntary/Mandatory)	Voluntary only; nonparticipation should not threaten economic viability of physician practices; must not favor participation of particular specialties, or groups of particular sizes or information technology (IT) capabilities; not linked to participation in other programs.	Not applicable.	Rewards for voluntary measurement and reporting; minimum number of encounters per patient per year; minimum number of patients/physician per year before data are considered valid.
Unit of Accountability	Physician practice groups and/or across health care systems (rather than individually) when feasible; no financial penalties based on factors outside of the physicians' control.	Physician office.	Develop methodology to allow physicians to receive payments for achieving systemwide Medicare savings attributable to individual physicians, physician group practices, or physician-guided chronic care coordination.
Improvement/ Excellence	Both.	Primary goal of pay for performance must be to promote continuously improving quality of care across the health care delivery system.	Reward both improving performance and meeting performance targets.
Weighting	Quality focused.	Data should be fully adjusted for case-mix composition.	Start with strongest weight for structural measures, followed by process measures and finally clinical outcome measures in a phased implementation.
Rewards/ Penalties	Rewards only.	Should be directed at positive rather than negative rewards.	Reward-based (positive incentives instead of withholds and penalties).

Absolute or Tournament	Absolute only (no comparative rankings).	In the early (i.e., reporting) stage, rewards should be absolute; as program progresses to pay based on actual performance, rewards should be balanced between rewarding high performance and rewarding substantial improvement over time.	Incentive payments should reward both performance improvement and meeting performance targets and not limited by tournament-type incentives.
Payment	Minimize potential financial and technological barriers, including costs of start-up; reimburse physicians for administrative costs.	Rewards must be greater than the cost of the physician's participation in a P4P program.	Financial rewards should cover administrative costs of participation and should increase proportionately based on the number of dimensions of care, time, and costs associated with documentation/IT.
Funding	New funds.	Ideally, new funds; if savings result, physicians should benefit from these savings; oppose withholds. However, due to the current fiscal environment, ACP recognizes that a redistribution of funds across and within geographic locations and specialties and between physicians and hospitals or other health care providers may be necessary.	New money and/or redistribution (e.g., from Part A); positive sustainable growth rate updates as a floor; no penalties for potential volume increases; support funds by setting aside a portion of the recommended inflation updates for 2006/7.
Phasing	Programs phased in to include all voluntary physicians (after pilot testing).	Supports incentives for IT—especially in the beginning for small practices.	Payment for structural (e.g., IT use) improvements, followed by payment for reporting, leading to payment for performance using validated measures (e.g., National Quality Forum [NQF], Ambulatory care Quality Alliance [AQA]).

continues

TABLE C-1 Continued

Design Issue	American Medical Association	American College of Physicians	American Academy of Family Physicians
Measure Development and Selection	Evidence-based; prospectively defined; allow for variation based on physician's patient-specific clinical judgment and patient preferences; developed collaboratively across specialties; risk-adjusted, stable for 2 years; aimed at areas with significant promise for improvement; pilot-tested, analyzing for patient de-selection; physicians review/comment on the accuracy and validity of both the data and analysis before use (see their preliminary ratings and adjust practice before public release).	Generally agrees with MedPAC; measures should be evidence-based, valid, and reliable; relevant to physician's clinical responsibilities; practical; relate to clinical conditions of highest priority; selected with stakeholder consensus.	Clinical measures validated by multi-stakeholder process, with full transparency; utilize valid peer groups, evidence-based statistical norms, and/or evidence-based clinical policies; incentives for adoption/utilization of IT, implementation of systems to improve quality of care and safety, access to timely care, patient acceptability and satisfaction with care.
Administrative vs. Chart Data	Both; medical record data collection must not be burdensome.	Does not support MedPAC's recommendation for submitting laboratory test values on claims. Chart abstraction data should be used only when the clinical/public health benefit clearly outweighs the burden and disruption of this kind of data collection.	Supports combination approach with phased implementation as described above and disclosure of data source(s) (e.g., administrative, chart audits, surveys, pharmacy).
Care Coordination	Encourage collaboration across all members of the health care team.	Fundamental reform of physician payment system needed; reimbursement should not be based on volume and episodes of acute illnesses, but on patient-centered, physician-guided care coordination and quality performance based on evidence-based clinical measures.	Supports care management fee for patient's chosen "personal medical home" and/or chronic care management fee for patients with selected chronic diseases.

TABLE C-2 Comparison Among Specialist Groups' Pay-for-Performance Position Statements

Design Issue	Alliance of Specialty Medicine	Society of Thoracic Surgeons	American College of Cardiology
Participation (Voluntary/Mandatory)	Voluntary through pilots.	Voluntary.	Not applicable.
Unit of Accountability	Not applicable.	Cardiac Thoracic surgeon group/hospital.	Physician groups rather than individual measurement; encourage collaboration between physician groups and across specialties (e.g., specialty and primary care groups).
Improvement/ Excellence	Not applicable.	Primary focus is on continuous quality improvement through compliance with process measures linked to quality and tracking of risk-adjusted outcome measures. Secondary focus is on achievement of excellence as defined by credible evidence-based thresholds for performance measures.	Excellence based on agreed-upon baseline standards.
Weighting	Not applicable.	Based on National Quality Forum (NQF) endorsed measures as either single measures or roll-up (composite) measures created with appropriate statistical modeling and risk adjustment for all outcome measures. Composite measures should include four domains of care: perioperative medical care, operative care, postoperative risk-adjusted mortality, and postoperative risk-adjusted morbidity.	Not applicable.

continues

TABLE C-2 Continued

Design Issue	Alliance of Specialty Medicine	Society of Thoracic Surgeons	American College of Cardiology
Rewards/ Penalties	Rewards only.	Rewards; no penalties. Rewards recognize continuous improvement in the quality of patient care and achievement of scientifically credible and achievable performance thresholds.	Rewards only.
Absolute or Tournament	Not applicable.	Absolute.	Absolute.
Payment	Not applicable.	Tiered incentive for achievement of structural, process, and risk-adjusted outcome measures. Advocates three phases: pay for participation in a clinical database, pay for demonstration of improvement over historical baselines, pay for performance through achievement of performance thresholds. Increased incentives for level of attainment of thresholds.	Rewards should correlate with investments made to improve care and sustainability of performance (e.g., time, training, technology).
Funding	New funds should be available if necessary.	Budget-neutral framework should not be tournament style (reducing all physician fees to create incentive pool), but should be based on shared savings generated through reductions in complications realized through continuous quality improvement and tracking of process measures linked to quality and risk-adjusted outcome measures.	Not applicable.

continues

Phasing	Should be phased in for physicians willing to participate.	Begin with payment for structural measures (pay for participation in a clinical database/pay for reporting) and move toward payment for process measures linked to quality and achievement of risk-adjusted outcome measures demonstrated to reduce costs. With feedback on performance, physicians should be encouraged to employ continuous quality improvement and engage in the creation of quality-focused cost containment.	Not applicable.
Measure Development and Selection	Evidence-based measures developed by physicians pertaining to issues that physicians can control; specialty specific; data collection and reporting should not be burdensome to practices.	Clinically relevant, scientifically valid and credible measures developed by physicians and their respective specialty societies. All measures should eventually be vetted through the NQF. Supports adoption of a consensus set of structural measures; process measures linked to quality and risk-adjusted outcome measures. Measures should be consistent with the principles and criteria recommended in the Institute of Medicine's 2006 *Performance Measurement* report. Attribution must be set to address systems of care and not individual physician measurement where appropriate.	Evidence-based and developed with a credible methodology. Risk-adjusted and clearly defined measures with consistent definitions; all data should be audited; providers should have the ability to comment on the data.

TABLE C-2 Continued

Design Issue	Alliance of Specialty Medicine	Society of Thoracic Surgeons	American College of Cardiology
Administrative vs. Chart Data	Supports the Centers for Medicare and Medicaid Services' (CMS) Physician Voluntary Reporting Program that uses administrative data.	Clinical data must be used to drive quality improvement. Administrative data should be linked to clinical data through a blending of specialty-specific databases and CMS financial data only to evaluate costs and efficiency, but not determine quality.	Chart data preferred over administrative data.
Care Coordination	Not applicable.	Encourages collaboration among providers and across disease conditions and care settings. Attribution (individual physician, physician group, hospital) must be appropriate in order to encourage effective hand-offs and transitions of care within and across episodes of care. Pay-for-performance programs must evaluate and reward systems of health care delivery.	Encourages collaboration among providers.

TABLE C-3 Comparison Among Purchaser and Consumer Groups' Pay-for-Performance Statements

Design Issue	Alliance of Community Health Plans	National Business Group on Health	National Patient Advocacy Foundation
Participation (Voluntary/ Mandatory)	Mandatory.	Voluntary	Voluntary.
Unit of Accountability	Health plans, physicians, hospitals, and other providers.	Not applicable.	Not applicable.
Improvement/ Excellence	Both; favors excellence.	Both.	Not applicable.
Weighting	Favors clinical performance.	Rewards specifically related to the quality of care provided, with a focus on efficiency.	Not applicable.
Rewards/ Penalties	Rewards.	Rewards.	Incentives that encourage improved quality of care delivery that will benefit both patients and providers; reimbursement systems should not be punitive.
Absolute or Tournament	Not applicable.	Not applicable.	Not applicable.
Payment	Not applicable.	Not applicable.	Allow provision for assisting physicians in obtaining the technology needed to participate.
Funding	New, dedicated stream of funding (add-on).	Not applicable.	Not applicable.

continues

TABLE C-3 Continued

Design Issue	Alliance of Community Health Plans	National Business Group on Health	National Patient Advocacy Foundation
Phasing	Start with Medicare Advantage plans and extend to physicians and hospitals (favor clinical).	Not applicable.	Not applicable.
Measure Development and Selection	Continue to evaluate Medicare plans; use evidence-based measures.	Performance measures should be incorporated in addition to structure and process measures; Medicare measures should be those developed by nationally recognized quality measurement organizations such as the National Committee for Quality Assurance or the National Quality Forum.	Not applicable.
Administrative vs. Chart Data	Both.	Possible financial assistance to providers and physicians in low-income urban areas to help with the purchase of software or systems needed.	Both, not to be overly burdensome or costly. In addition include interoperable electronic health infrastructures.
Care Coordination	Support care coordination (MedPAC).	Care coordination, hand-offs, and the team approach should be a part of pay for performance and measured appropriately, rather than solely single practitioners or facilities being measured for their portion of the treatment of an episode of care.	Collaboration among all stakeholders to include participation from the patient, physician and provider communities.

TABLE C-4 Ambulatory care Quality Alliance

Design Issues	Ambulatory care Quality Alliance (AQA)[a]
Participation (Voluntary/Mandatory)	Voluntary.
Unit of Accountability	Physicians and physician groups.
Improvement/Excellence	Not applicable.
Weighting	Alignment or linkage of quality and cost of care measures.
Rewards/Penalties	Not applicable.
Absolute or Tournament	Not applicable.
Payment	Not applicable.
Funding	Not applicable.
Phasing	No discussion to date.
Measure Development and Selection	AQA does not develop measures; it approves measures developed by National Committee for Quality Assurance, Joint Commission on Accreditation of Healthcare Organizations, American Medical Association PCPI, and other medical specialty organizations that meet AQA-defined parameters.
Administrative vs. Chart Data	Implementation of measures should be as least burdensome as possible. While the AQA Performance Measurement Workgroup acknowledges that administrative data should be considered as the logical starting point, there is interest in moving beyond claims and other administrative data as soon as is practicable. As appropriate, measures derived from medical chart review should not be excluded.
Care Coordination	Not applicable.

[a]The AQA does not specifically address or take a position on pay-for-performance programs; rather, its work focuses on evidence-based, valid, reliable performance measures for quality improvement and accountability. AQA encourages implementation of standardized performance measures endorsed by AQA for physician assessment, one component of which may be pay-for-performance programs.

D

MedPAC Data Runs

As requested in its congressional mandate, the committee consulted with the Medicare Payment Advisory Committee (MedPAC) in its examination of pay for performance. Specifically, MedPAC was requested by the committee to perform some limited data runs on payments associated with the treatment of three clinical conditions: coronary artery disease, chronic heart failure, and diabetes. The following tables represent data submitted to the committee by MedPAC and include breakdowns of payments by condition, as well as aggregations for those beneficiaries who were treated for more than one of the three conditions. Additionally, the data include the number of unique physician identification numbers (UPINs) submitting claims per beneficiary, as well as the types of claims (evaluation and management, major surgery, other surgery, testing, and imaging).

These data were generated from the Medicare 5 percent Standard Analytic Files for 2003 (inpatient, outpatient, and physician/supplier). Beneficiaries living in the U.S. territories are not counted in this analysis, but beneficiaries under the age of 65 and those with claims from managed care and hospice care, decedents, and new entrants are included.

These data helped inform the committee as to the nature of the care being delivered to Medicare beneficiaries and the payments associated with this care. The committee used the data to derive conclusions regarding the attribution of care and the magnitude of potential reward levels.

TABLE D-1 Number of Beneficiaries and Payments for Beneficiaries in Groups A–G

Group	(a) Number of Beneficiaries	(b) Total Payments (Inpatient, Outpatient, and Carrier)	(c) Total Physician Payments	(d) Total Physician Fee Schedule Payments	(e) Total Physician Fee Schedule Payments with Condition
A—Diabetes, Chronic Heart Failure, & Coronary Artery Disease	33,156	$930,459,017.78	$190,763,248.74	$145,289,007.75	$63,478,717.18
B—Chronic Heart Failure & Coronary Artery Disease; not Diabetes	45,669	$973,068,755.23	$204,803,139.36	$156,203,604.11	$51,811,091.99
C—Chronic Heart Failure & Diabetes; not Coronary Artery Disease	20,084	$343,667,332.55	$77,771,058.17	$57,876,926.78	$17,685,633.11
D—Diabetes & Coronary Artery Disease; not Chronic Heart Failure	52,831	$650,379,010.79	$180,745,583.66	$135,706,435.84	$49,925,585.96
E—Chronic Heart Failure; not Diabetes & Coronary Artery Disease	44,624	$571,843,797.98	$133,677,894.22	$98,210,007.62	$15,564,360.34
F—Coronary Artery Disease; not Diabetes & Chronic Heart Failure	139,998	$1,278,200,988.51	$388,080,620.15	$290,563,134.95	$73,437,377.10
G—Diabetes; not Chronic Heart Failure & Coronary Artery Disease	183,021	$1,010,989,783.78	$358,203,918.84	$254,121,712.13	$58,724,822.67
X—No Condition Category Assigned	1,108,039	$3,659,514,615.32	$1,484,938,239.88	$1,038,689,792.23	
Total in Groups	519,383	$5,758,608,686.62	$1,534,045,463.14	$1,137,970,829.18	$330,627,588.35
Total in File	1,627,422	$9,418,123,301.94	$3,018,983,703.02	$2,176,660,621.41	$330,627,588.35

NOTES:
Claim lines with invalid provider numbers have been removed from the physician file for all tables.
(a) All beneficiaries with at least one claim line with a valid provider number.
(b) Payments from the inpatient, outpatient, and carrier file.
(c) Carrier file in total, regardless of provider type and fee schedule designation.
(d) Carrier file, only payments associated with the fee schedule.
(e) Carrier file, payments associated with the fee schedule for the condition associated with the disease group.

TABLE D-2 Number of Physician Providers per Beneficiary in
Groups A–G

	(a)	(b)	(c)
Group	Sum Number of Physician UPINs per Beneficiary	Mean Number of Physician UPINs per Beneficiary	Median Number of Physician UPINs per Beneficiary
A—Diabetes, Chronic Heart Failure, & Coronary Artery Disease	433,829	13.3919	12
B—Chronic Heart Failure & Coronary Artery Disease; not Diabetes	500,679	11.2215	10
C—Chronic Heart Failure & Diabetes; not Coronary Artery Disease	181,513	9.2689	8
D—Diabetes & Coronary Artery Disease; not Chronic Heart Failure	417,751	8.0997	7
E—Chronic Heart Failure; not Diabetes & Coronary Artery Disease	337,732	7.7802	6
F—Coronary Artery Disease; not Diabetes & Chronic Heart Failure	953,450	6.9683	6
G—Diabetes; not Chronic Heart Failure & Coronary Artery Disease	884,283	4.9764	4
X—No Condition Category Assigned	4,118,603	3.9818	3
Total in Groups	3,681,210	7.2764	6
Total in File	7,730,303	5.0191	4

NOTES:
Claim lines with invalid provider numbers have been removed from the physician file for all tables.
Carrier file data only.
Outliers above 99 percent have been removed. Outlier threshold is calculated for each group and in total, therefore, the "Total in File" and "Total in Groups" will not equate to the sum of the groups.
Only physician providers are included in this analysis. Physician provider designation is based on HCFA specialty code.
(a)–(g) Carrier file; physician providers; regardless of condition.
(h) Carrier file; physician providers; condition related claims only.

(d) Maximum Number of Physician UPINs per Beneficiary	(e) Standard Deviation Number of Physician UPINs per Beneficiary	(f) Total Number of Beneficiaries	(g) Total Number of UPINs	(h) Total Number of UPINs Related to Condition
44	8	33,156	174,016	100,639
38	7	45,669	190,398	85,129
36	7	20,084	116,830	54,526
29	5	52,831	187,777	93,058
30	6	44,624	171,838	55,812
24	4	139,998	262,774	89,953
21	4	183,021	285,479	135,033
16	3	1,108,039	389,895	
30	5	519,383	363,096	212,855
23	4	1,627,422	406,984	

TABLE D-3 Proportion of Beneficiaries with 1–10+ Physicians Billing for Care

Group	(a) Total Beneficiaries w/ Physician Providers	(b) 1 Physician UPIN per Beneficiary	(c) 2–5 Physician UPINs per Beneficiary	(d) 6–9 Physician UPINs per Beneficiary	(e) 10+ Physician UPINs per Beneficiary
A—Diabetes, Chronic Heart Failure, & Coronary Artery Disease	32,395	0.96%	14.14%	23.36%	61.54%
B—Chronic Heart Failure & Coronary Artery Disease; not Diabetes	44,618	2.01%	20.13%	26.33%	51.53%
C—Chronic Heart Failure & Diabetes; not Coronary Artery Disease	19,583	4.22%	29.95%	27.39%	38.44%
D—Diabetes & Coronary Artery Disease; not Chronic Heart Failure	51,576	2.99%	33.94%	31.84%	31.23%
E—Chronic Heart Failure; not Diabetes & Coronary Artery Disease	43,409	6.87%	35.76%	27.42%	29.95%
F—Coronary Artery Disease; not Diabetes & Chronic Heart Failure	136,826	4.70%	40.07%	31.75%	23.48%
G—Diabetes; not Chronic Heart Failure & Coronary Artery Disease	177,694	11.25%	55.46%	22.35%	10.94%
X—No Condition Category Assigned	1,034,357	19.90%	56.42%	17.73%	5.94%
Total in Groups	505,912	6.52%	40.69%	26.91%	25.88%
Total in File	1,540,183	15.51%	51.26%	20.75%	12.49%

NOTES:
Claim lines with invalid provider numbers have been removed from the physician file for all tables.
Carrier file data only.
Outliers above 99 percent have been removed.
Outlier threshold is calculated for each group and in total, therefore, the "Total in File" and "Total in Groups" will not equate to the sum of the groups.
Only physician providers are included in this analysis. Physician provider designation is based on Health Care Financing Administration specialty code.

TABLE D-4 Proportion of Beneficiaries Associated with a Percent of Physician Provider Payments Allocated to One Provider

Group	(a) Total Beneficiaries w/ Physician Providers	(b) 70–100% of Payments to Provider	(c) 50–69% of Payments to Provider	(d) 35–49% of Payments to Provider	(e) 20–34% of Payments to Provider	(f) 0–19% of Payments to Provider
A—Diabetes, Chronic Heart Failure, & Coronary Artery Disease	32,395	7.93%	16.70%	27.14%	37.67%	10.55%
B—Chronic Heart Failure & Coronary Artery Disease; not Diabetes	44,618	11.28%	18.86%	28.39%	33.97%	7.51%
C—Chronic Heart Failure & Diabetes; not Coronary Artery Disease	19,583	17.11%	21.43%	26.98%	28.52%	5.96%
D—Diabetes & Coronary Artery Disease; not Chronic Heart Failure	51,576	15.93%	24.47%	30.28%	25.98%	3.33%
E—Chronic Heart Failure; not Diabetes & Coronary Artery Disease	43,409	21.61%	22.61%	26.14%	25.14%	4.51%
F—Coronary Artery Disease; not Diabetes & Chronic Heart Failure	136,826	20.59%	25.83%	29.18%	21.96%	2.42%
G—Diabetes; not Chronic Heart Failure & Coronary Artery Disease	177,694	31.20%	27.71%	24.75%	14.68%	1.66%
X—No Condition Category Assigned	1,034,357	38.66%	25.71%	20.48%	10.61%	4.54%
Total in Groups	505,912	22.17%	24.72%	27.23%	22.43%	3.44%
Total in File	1,540,183	33.26%	25.41%	22.73%	14.50%	4.10%

NOTES:
Claim lines with invalid provider numbers have been removed from the physician file for all tables.
Carrier file data only.
Outliers above 99 percent have been removed.
Outlier threshold is calculated for each group and in total, therefore, the "Total in File" and "Total in Groups" will not equate to the sum of the groups. Only physician providers are included in this analysis. Physician provider designation is based on Health Care Financing Administration specialty code.
The beneficiary is counted once in the highest provider category.

TABLE D-5 Proportion of Beneficiaries Associated with a Percent of Physician Provider Payments Allocated to One Provider for the Condition

Group	(a) Total Beneficiaries w/ Physician Providers	(b) 70–100% of Payments to Provider	(c) 50–69% of Payments to Provider	(d) 35–49% of Payments to Provider	(e) 20–34% of Payments to Provider	(f) 0–19% of Payments to Provider
A—Diabetes, Chronic Heart Failure, & Coronary Artery Disease	32,225	22.11%	27.09%	28.26%	20.06%	2.48%
B—Chronic Heart Failure & Coronary Artery Disease; not Diabetes	43,652	38.42%	28.40%	21.24%	10.79%	1.15%
C—Chronic Heart Failure & Diabetes; not Coronary Artery Disease	19,173	43.67%	27.13%	18.69%	9.46%	1.05%
D—Diabetes & Coronary Artery Disease; not Chronic Heart Failure	50,844	41.55%	32.17%	19.33%	6.40%	0.54%
E—Chronic Heart Failure; not Diabetes & Coronary Artery Disease	38,728	67.81%	18.59%	8.56%	3.49%	1.55%
F—Coronary Artery Disease; not Diabetes & Chronic Heart Failure	128,289	68.20%	21.93%	6.78%	1.51%	1.57%
G—Diabetes; not Chronic Heart Failure & Coronary Artery Disease	169,507	68.97%	21.18%	6.84%	1.61%	1.40%
Total in Groups	482,071	59.03%	23.67%	11.47%	4.48%	1.35%
Total in File	473,080	59.85%	23.72%	11.14%	4.00%	1.29%

NOTES:
Claim lines with invalid provider numbers have been removed from the physician file for all tables.
Carrier file data only; condition related.
Outliers above 99 percent have been removed.
Outlier threshold is calculated for each group and in total, therefore, the "Total in File" and "Total in Groups" will not equate to the sum of the groups.
Only physician providers are included in this analysis. Physician provider designation is based on HCFA specialty code.
The beneficiary is counted once in the highest provider category.

TABLE D-6 Proportion of Beneficiaries Associated with a Percent of Physician Provider Claims Allocated to One Provider

Group	(a) Total Beneficiaries w/ Physician Providers	(b) 70–100% of Claims to Provider	(c) 50–69% of Claims to Provider	(d) 35–49% of Claims to Provider	(e) 20–34% of Claims to Provider	(f) 0–19% of Claims to Provider
A—Diabetes, Chronic Heart Failure, & Coronary Artery Disease	32,395	6.24%	16.31%	23.24%	37.84%	16.37%
B—Chronic Heart Failure & Coronary Artery Disease; not Diabetes	44,618	8.90%	18.53%	23.51%	35.89%	13.17%
C—Chronic Heart Failure & Diabetes; not Coronary Artery Disease	19,583	16.05%	22.89%	22.64%	29.42%	8.99%
D—Diabetes & Coronary Artery Disease; not Chronic Heart Failure	51,576	11.88%	23.14%	26.31%	32.03%	6.64%
E—Chronic Heart Failure; not Diabetes & Coronary Artery Disease	43,409	19.75%	24.23%	21.37%	27.15%	7.49%
F—Coronary Artery Disease; not Diabetes & Chronic Heart Failure	136,826	14.47%	24.46%	25.30%	30.56%	5.21%
G—Diabetes; not Chronic Heart Failure & Coronary Artery Disease	177,694	28.96%	30.22%	20.48%	18.09%	2.25%
X—No Condition Category Assigned	1,034,357	33.27%	30.74%	17.47%	17.08%	1.44%
Total in Groups	505,912	18.80%	25.24%	23.00%	26.97%	5.99%
Total in File	1,540,183	28.52%	28.95%	19.32%	20.36%	2.85%

NOTES:
Claim lines with invalid provider numbers have been removed from the physician file for all tables.
Carrier file data only.
Outliers above 99 percent have been removed.
Outlier threshold is calculated for each group and in total, therefore, the "Total in File" and "Total in Groups" will not equate to the sum of the groups.
Only physician providers are included in this analysis. Physician provider designation is based on HCFA specialty code.
The beneficiary is counted once in the highest provider category.

TABLE D-7 Proportion of Beneficiaries Associated with a Percent of Physician Provider Claims Allocated to One Provider for the Condition

Group	(a) Total Beneficiaries w/ Physician Providers	(b) 70–100% of Claims to Provider	(c) 50–69% of Claims to Provider	(d) 35–49% of Claims to Provider	(e) 20–34% of Claims to Provider	(f) 0–19% of Claims to Provider
A—Diabetes, Chronic Heart Failure, & Coronary Artery Disease	32,225	18.30%	27.43%	22.56%	26.33%	5.38%
B—Chronic Heart Failure & Coronary Artery Disease; not Diabetes	43,652	29.84%	29.84%	16.79%	20.61%	2.93%
C—Chronic Heart Failure & Diabetes; not Coronary Artery Disease	19,173	41.46%	29.30%	13.73%	13.86%	1.65%
D—Diabetes & Coronary Artery Disease; not Chronic Heart Failure	50,844	34.28%	34.82%	16.74%	13.13%	1.04%
E—Chronic Heart Failure; not Diabetes & Coronary Artery Disease	38,728	59.70%	24.09%	5.29%	10.08%	0.84%
F—Coronary Artery Disease; not Diabetes & Chronic Heart Failure	128,289	54.73%	30.54%	6.50%	7.77%	0.46%

G—Diabetes; not Chronic Heart Failure & Coronary Artery Disease	169,507	68.24%	23.79%	4.23%	3.61%	0.13%
Total in Groups	482,071	52.63%	27.87%	8.97%	9.60%	0.93%
Total in File	473,080	53.44%	28.06%	8.77%	9.02%	0.72%

NOTES:
Claim lines with invalid provider numbers have been removed from the physician file for all tables.
Carrier file data only; condition related.
Outliers above 99 percent have been removed.
Outlier threshold is calculated for each group and in total, therefore, the "Total in File" and "Total in Groups" will not equate to the sum of the groups.
Only physician providers are included in this analysis. Physician provider designation is based on HCFA specialty code.
The beneficiary is counted once in the highest provider category.

TABLE D-8 Payments by Type of Service for Beneficiaries Within Groups

Group	(a) Evaluation & Management— Payment ($)	(b) Evaluation & Management— Percent
A—Diabetes, Chronic Heart Failure, & Coronary Artery Disease	86,471,514	45%
B—Chronic Heart Failure & Coronary Artery Disease; not Diabetes	91,924,988	45%
C—Chronic Heart Failure & Diabetes; not Coronary Artery Disease	36,190,515	47%
D—Diabetes & Coronary Artery Disease; not Chronic Heart Failure	64,463,785	36%
E—Chronic Heart Failure; not Diabetes & Coronary Artery Disease	60,720,321	45%
F—Coronary Artery Disease; not Diabetes & Chronic Heart Failure	130,330,105	34%
G—Diabetes; not Chronic Heart Failure & Coronary Artery Disease	132,909,072	37%
X—No Condition Category Assigned	500,560,122	34%
Total in Groups	603,010,300	39%
Total in File	1,103,570,422	37%

(c) Major Procedure— Payment ($)	(d) Major Procedure— Percent	(e) Other Procedure— Payment ($)	(f) Other Procedure— Percent	(g) Testing— Payment ($)	(h) Testing Percent
19,163,429	10%	25,373,801	13%	12,051,707	6%
21,282,956	10%	24,885,905	12%	12,995,751	6%
4,853,795	6%	11,645,941	15%	5,219,937	7%
19,128,346	11%	32,277,301	18%	15,187,808	8%
8,747,398	7%	18,423,696	14%	8,624,945	6%
40,659,972	10%	70,003,113	18%	30,908,776	8%
18,909,673	5%	79,599,074	22%	32,043,053	9%
78,532,780	5%	355,184,517	24%	114,339,344	8%
132,745,569	9%	262,208,831	17%	117,031,976	8%
211,278,349	7%	617,393,349	20%	231,371,321	8%

continues

TABLE D-8 Continued

Group	(i) Imaging— Payment ($)	(j) Imaging— Percent	(k) Durable Medical Equipment— Payment ($)
A—Diabetes, Chronic Heart Failure, & Coronary Artery Disease	18,813,256	10%	32,163
B—Chronic Heart Failure & Coronary Artery Disease; not Diabetes	23,283,835	11%	14,252
C—Chronic Heart Failure & Diabetes; not Coronary Artery Disease	7,044,547	9%	16,958
D—Diabetes & Coronary Artery Disease; not Chronic Heart Failure	26,396,528	15%	30,039
E—Chronic Heart Failure; not Diabetes & Coronary Artery Disease	13,824,528	10%	11,321
F—Coronary Artery Disease; not Diabetes & Chronic Heart Failure	65,119,481	17%	52,823
G—Diabetes; not Chronic Heart Failure & Coronary Artery Disease	38,948,223	11%	116,824
X—No Condition Category Assigned	186,770,390	13%	392,111
Total in Groups	193,430,400	13%	274,380
Total in File	380,200,790	13%	666,491

NOTES:
Claim lines with invalid provider numbers have been removed from the physician file for all tables.
Carrier file data only.

(l) Durable Medical Equipment— Percent	(m) Other— Payment ($)	(n) Other— Percent	(o) Exceptions and Unclassified— Payment ($)	(p) Exceptions and Unclassified— Percent	(q) Total Payments ($)
0%	28,039,940	15%	817,439	0%	190,763,249
0%	29,533,420	14%	882,031	0%	204,803,139
0%	12,380,993	16%	418,372	1%	77,771,058
0%	22,594,208	13%	667,568	0%	180,745,584
0%	22,479,758	17%	845,928	1%	133,677,894
0%	49,551,807	13%	1,454,542	0%	388,080,620
0%	54,017,297	15%	1,660,703	0%	358,203,919
0%	241,534,417	16%	7,624,558	1%	1,484,938,240
0%	218,597,423	14%	6,746,583	0%	1,534,045,463
0%	460,131,841	15%	14,371,140	0%	3,018,983,703

TABLE D-9 Average Parts A & B Enrollment by Beneficiary Designation

(a) Class	(b) Total Months	(c) Beneficiaries	(d) Average Months
Total	24,110,216	2,110,869	11.42
Over 65	20,642,413	1,803,117	11.45
Disabled	3,418,342	303,270	11.27
ESRD	206,976	19,445	10.64
Hospice	281,438	36,306	7.75
Medicare Advantage	3,333,810	287,241	11.61
Deceased	627,655	96,879	6.48
Entered	898,723	131,829	6.82

NOTES:
Enrolled in either Part A or Part B.
Classifications are not mutually exclusive. A beneficiary can be in more than one class.

TABLE D-10 Preventive Services

Service	Total Carrier File Payments	Associated Beneficiaries
GI Tract Work-up After Initial Diagnosis of Iron Deficiency Anemia	$1,908,370.72	8,239
Breast Cancer Screening	$15,871,566.27	245,365
Total	$17,779,936.99	253,604

NOTES:
There were 1151 beneficiaries with both iron deficiency anemia and breast cancer.
Payments include all claims from the carrier file regardless of physician provider or fee-schedule designation.
ACEPRO Analysis had a more limited population and resulted in 208,341 benes for breast cancer screening and 5,977 for iron deficiency anemia.

TABLE D-11 Vaccine Payments

Vaccination Type	Total Carrier File Payments
Total	$11,788,264.27
Influenza	$1,841,885.65
Pneumococcal	$9,946,378.62

NOTES:
Payments include all claims from the carrier file regardless of physician provider or fee-schedule designation.
Pneumococcal vaccine included CPT codes 90658, 90660, and G0008.
Influenza vaccine included CPT codes 90732 and G0009.

TABLE D-12 Evaluation and Management Claims—Proportion of Beneficiaries with 1–10+ Physicians Billing for Care

Group	Total Beneficiaries w/ Physician Providers	1 Physician UPIN per Beneficiary	2–5 Physician UPINs per Beneficiary	Less than 5 Physician UPINs per Beneficiary	6–9 Physician UPINs per Beneficiary	10+ Physician UPINs per Beneficiary
A—Diabetes, Chronic Heart Failure, & Coronary Artery Disease	32,755	1.43%	22.60%	24.03%	28.50%	47.47%
B—Chronic Heart Failure & Coronary Artery Disease; not Diabetes	44,850	2.79%	30.02%	32.81%	30.56%	36.64%
C—Chronic Heart Failure & Diabetes; not Coronary Artery Disease	19,784	5.49%	39.67%	45.17%	27.56%	27.28%
D—Diabetes & Coronary Artery Disease; not Chronic Heart Failure	52,230	4.13%	46.59%	50.72%	30.77%	18.51%
E—Chronic Heart Failure; not Diabetes & Coronary Artery Disease	43,610	8.93%	44.87%	53.80%	26.44%	19.76%
F—Coronary Artery Disease; not Diabetes & Chronic Heart Failure	137,709	6.73%	52.87%	59.60%	27.88%	12.52%
G—Diabetes; not Chronic Heart Failure & Coronary Artery Disease	180,054	14.18%	61.81%	75.98%	17.79%	6.22%
X—No Condition Category Assigned	1,016,725	24.06%	59.87%	83.93%	13.22%	2.85%
Total in File	1,529,789	18.84%	56.57%	75.42%	17.06%	7.53%
Total in Groups	510,910	8.54%	50.25%	58.79%	24.76%	16.45%

NOTES:
Claim lines with invalid provider numbers have been removed from the physician file for all tables.
Carrier file data only.
Outliers above 99 percent have been removed.
Outlier threshold is calculated for each group and in total, therefore, the "Total in File" and "Total in Groups" will not equate to the sum of the groups.
Only physician providers are included in this analysis. Physician provider designation is based on HCFA specialty code.

TABLE D-13 Evaluation and Management Claims—Proportion of Beneficiaries Associated with a Percent of Physician Provider Payments Allocated to One Provider

Group	Total Beneficiaries w/Physician Providers	70–100% of Payments to Provider	50–69% of Payments to Provider	35–49% of Payments to Provider	More than 35% of Payments to Providers	20–34% of Payments to Provider
A—Diabetes, Chronic Heart Failure, & Coronary Artery Disease	32,755	7.41%	15.73%	25.76%	48.90%	37.85%
B—Chronic Heart Failure & Coronary Artery Disease; not Diabetes	44,850	10.45%	18.46%	27.34%	56.24%	34.30%
C—Chronic Heart Failure & Diabetes; not Coronary Artery Disease	19,784	17.56%	21.68%	25.93%	65.16%	28.14%
D—Diabetes & Coronary Artery Disease; not Chronic Heart Failure	52,230	13.23%	21.39%	29.56%	64.19%	30.36%
E—Chronic Heart Failure; not Diabetes & Coronary Artery Disease	43,610	21.69%	22.88%	25.37%	69.94%	24.98%
F—Coronary Artery Disease; not Diabetes & Chronic Heart Failure	137,709	17.20%	23.19%	28.71%	69.10%	26.65%
G—Diabetes; not Chronic Heart Failure &x Coronary Artery Disease	180,054	29.74%	27.65%	24.09%	81.47%	15.88%
X—No Condition Category Assigned	1,016,725	34.44%	24.98%	19.93%	79.35%	12.20%
Total in File	1,529,789	29.70%	24.50%	22.13%	76.33%	16.42%
Total in Groups	510,910	20.39%	23.61%	26.48%	70.48%	24.58%

NOTES:
Claim lines with invalid provider numbers have been removed from the physician file for all tables.
Carrier file data only.
Outliers above 99 percent have been removed.
Outlier threshold is calculated for each group and in total, therefore, the "Total in File" and "Total in Groups" will not equate to the sum of the groups.
Only physician providers are included in this analysis. Physician provider designation is based on HCFA specialty code.
The beneficiary is counted once in the highest provider category.

TABLE D-14 Evaluation and Management Claims for Beneficiaries with Hospitalization—Proportion of Beneficiaries with 1–10+ Physicians Billing for Care

Group	Total Beneficiaries w/ Physician Providers	1 Physician UPIN per Beneficiary	2–5 Physician UPINs per Beneficiary	Less than 5 Physician UPINs per Beneficiary	6–9 Physician UPINs per Beneficiary	10+ Physician UPINs per Beneficiary
A—Diabetes, Chronic Heart Failure, & Coronary Artery Disease	27,991	0.67%	16.62%	17.29%	28.52%	54.19%
B—Chronic Heart Failure & Coronary Artery Disease; not Diabetes	35,523	1.07%	21.28%	22.35%	32.60%	45.05%
C—Chronic Heart Failure & Diabetes; not Coronary Artery Disease	13,119	1.49%	26.88%	28.37%	32.35%	39.28%
D—Diabetes & Coronary Artery Disease; not Chronic Heart Failure	26,155	1.19%	28.29%	29.48%	37.00%	33.52%
E—Chronic Heart Failure; not Diabetes & Coronary Artery Disease	25,536	1.89%	31.18%	33.07%	34.49%	32.44%
F—Coronary Artery Disease; not Diabetes & Chronic Heart Failure	56,770	1.47%	32.77%	34.23%	38.89%	26.88%
G—Diabetes; not Chronic Heart Failure & Coronary Artery Disease	39,281	2.18%	35.73%	37.91%	36.24%	25.86%
X—No Condition Category Assigned	144,518	2.79%	41.30%	44.09%	35.50%	20.41%
Total in File	368,810	1.97%	33.46%	35.44%	35.23%	29.34%
Total in Groups	224,284	1.45%	28.42%	29.86%	35.05%	35.09%

NOTES:
Claim lines with invalid provider numbers have been removed from the physician file for all tables.
Carrier file data only.
Outliers above 99 percent have been removed.
Outlier threshold is calculated for each group and in total, therefore, the "Total in File" and "Total in Groups" will not equate to the sum of the groups.
Only physician providers are included in this analysis. Physician provider designation is based on HCFA specialty code.

TABLE D-15 Evaluation and Management Claims for Beneficiaries with Hospitalization—Proportion of Beneficiaries Associated with a Percent of Physician Provider Payments Allocated to One Provider

Group	Total Beneficiaries w/ Physician Providers	70–100% of Payments to Provider	50–69% of Payments to Provider	35–49% of Payments to Provider	More than 35% of Payments to Providers	20–34% of Payments to Provider
A—Diabetes, Chronic Heart Failure, & Coronary Artery Disease	27,991	5.40%	14.18%	24.97%	44.55%	40.33%
B—Chronic Heart Failure & Coronary Artery Disease; not Diabetes	35,523	6.67%	15.92%	27.32%	49.91%	38.52%
C—Chronic Heart Failure & Diabetes; not Coronary Artery Disease	13,119	9.72%	18.55%	27.01%	55.27%	35.16%
D—Diabetes & Coronary Artery Disease; not Chronic Heart Failure	26,155	6.37%	16.03%	28.65%	51.05%	39.29%
E—Chronic Heart Failure; not Diabetes & Coronary Artery Disease	25,536	10.44%	19.67%	28.01%	58.12%	34.21%
F—Coronary Artery Disease; not Diabetes & Chronic Heart Failure	56,770	7.26%	17.41%	29.75%	54.42%	37.99%
G—Diabetes; not Chronic Heart Failure & Coronary Artery Disease	39,281	10.08%	19.82%	29.83%	59.73%	33.59%
X—No Condition Category Assigned	144,518	11.59%	21.19%	29.72%	62.50%	32.09%
Total in File	368,810	9.31%	18.86%	28.86%	57.03%	35.20%
Total in Groups	224,284	7.83%	17.37%	28.31%	53.51%	37.16%

NOTES:

Claim lines with invalid provider numbers have been removed from the physician file for all tables.

Carrier file data only.

Outliers above 99 percent have been removed.

Outlier threshold is calculated for each group and in total, therefore, the "Total in File" and "Total in Groups" will not equate to the sum of the groups.

Only physician providers are included in this analysis. Physician provider designation is based on HCFA specialty code.

The beneficiary is counted once in the highest provider category.

TABLE D-16 Evaluation and Management Claims for Beneficiaries without Hospitalization—Proportion of Beneficiaries with 1–10+ Physicians Billing for Care

Group	Total Beneficiaries w/ Physician Providers	Total Benes not Hospitalized/ total Benes (from Table 1)	1 Physician UPIN per Beneficiary	2–5 Physician UPINs per Beneficiary	Less than 5 Physician UPINs per Beneficiary	6–9 Physician UPINs per Beneficiary	10+ Physician UPINs per Beneficiary
A—Diabetes, Chronic Heart Failure, & Coronary Artery Disease	4,751	14.50%	5.87%	57.90%	63.78%	28.44%	7.79%
B—Chronic Heart Failure Coronary Artery Disease; not Diabetes	9,303	20.74%	9.35%	63.49%	72.84%	22.81%	4.35%
C—Chronic Heart Failure & Diabetes; not Coronary Artery Disease	6,661	33.67%	13.38%	64.90%	78.28%	18.14%	3.59%
D—Diabetes & Coronary Artery Disease; not Chronic Heart Failure	26,081	49.93%	7.07%	64.94%	72.01%	24.52%	3.47%
E—Chronic Heart Failure; not Diabetes & Coronary Artery Disease	18,093	41.49%	18.84%	64.15%	82.99%	15.06%	1.95%
F—Coronary Artery Disease; not Diabetes & Chronic Heart Failure	80,628	58.55%	10.47%	67.23%	77.70%	20.23%	2.07%
G—Diabetes; not Chronic Heart Failure & Coronary Artery Disease	140,725	78.16%	17.53%	69.11%	86.64%	12.65%	0.71%
X—No Condition Category Assigned	872,733	85.84%	27.57%	62.91%	90.48%	9.52%	
Total in File	1,161,313	75.91%	24.20%	63.90%	88.09%	11.28%	0.63%
Total in Groups	286,237	56.02%	14.12%	67.42%	81.54%	16.74%	1.73%

NOTES:

Claim lines with invalid provider numbers have been removed from the physician file for all tables.

Carrier file data only.

Outliers above 99 percent have been removed.

Outlier threshold is calculated for each group and in total, therefore, the "Total in File" and "Total in Groups" will not equate to the sum of the groups. Physician provider designation is based on HCFA specialty code.

Only physician providers are included in this analysis. Physician provider designation is based on HCFA specialty code.

TABLE D-17 Evaluation and Management Claims for Beneficiaries without Hospitalization—Proportion of Beneficiaries Associated with a Percent of Physician Provider Payments Allocated to One Provider

Group	Total Beneficiaries w/ Physician Providers	70–100% of Payments to Provider	50–69% of Payments to Provider	35–49% of Payments to Provider	More than 35% of Payments to Providers	20–34% of Payments to Provider
A—Diabetes, Chronic Heart Failure, & Coronary Artery Disease	4,751	19.24%	24.92%	30.46%	74.62%	23.05%
B—Chronic Heart Failure & Coronary Artery Disease; not Diabetes	9,303	24.90%	28.20%	27.40%	80.49%	18.03%
C—Chronic Heart Failure & Diabetes; not Coronary Artery Disease	6,661	33.00%	27.86%	23.71%	84.57%	14.07%
D—Diabetes & Coronary Artery Disease; not Chronic Heart Failure	26,081	20.10%	26.74%	30.42%	77.26%	21.26%
E—Chronic Heart Failure; not Diabetes & Coronary Artery Disease	18,093	37.54%	27.38%	21.61%	86.53%	11.82%
F—Coronary Artery Disease; not Diabetes & Chronic Heart Failure	80,628	24.27%	27.33%	28.00%	79.60%	18.51%
G—Diabetes; not Chronic Heart Failure & Coronary Artery Disease	140,725	35.23%	29.84%	22.43%	87.50%	10.82%
X—No Condition Category Assigned	872,733	38.20%	25.59%	18.29%	82.08%	8.82%
Total in File	1,161,313	36.17%	26.27%	19.94%	82.38%	10.35%
Total in Groups	286,237	30.26%	28.51%	25.00%	83.77%	14.54%

NOTES:
Claim lines with invalid provider numbers have been removed from the physician file for all tables.
Carrier file data only.
Outliers above 99 percent have been removed.
Outlier threshold is calculated for each group and in total, therefore, the "Total in File" and "Total in Groups" will not equate to the sum of the groups.
Only physician providers are included in this analysis. Physician provider designation is based on HCFA specialty code.
The beneficiary is counted once in the highest provider category.

TABLE D-18 Evaluation and Management Claims Excluding Place of Service 21—Proportion of Beneficiaries with 1–10+ Physicians Billing for Care

Group	Total Beneficiaries w/ Physician Providers	1 Physician UPIN per Beneficiary	2–5 Physician UPINs per Beneficiary	Less than 5 Physician UPINs per Beneficiary	6–9 Physician UPINs per Beneficiary	10+ Physician UPINs per Beneficiary
A—Diabetes, Chronic Heart Failure, & Coronary Artery Disease	32,545	3.28%	42.82%	46.09%	37.11%	16.80%
B—Chronic Heart Failure & Coronary Artery Disease; not Diabetes	44,347	5.17%	50.55%	55.72%	32.79%	11.49%
C—Chronic Heart Failure & Diabetes; not Coronary Artery Disease	19,586	8.06%	57.62%	65.68%	26.81%	7.52%
D—Diabetes & Coronary Artery Disease; not Chronic Heart Failure	52,038	5.35%	57.14%	62.49%	29.90%	7.61%
E—Chronic Heart Failure; not Diabetes & Coronary Artery Disease	43,012	12.20%	60.68%	72.88%	22.45%	4.67%
F—Coronary Artery Disease; not Diabetes & Chronic Heart Failure	137,266	7.91%	61.31%	69.22%	25.81%	4.97%
G—Diabetes; not Chronic Heart Failure & Coronary Artery Disease	179,095	15.06%	66.60%	81.66%	16.42%	1.92%
X—No Condition Category Assigned	1,013,335	24.79%	62.48%	87.26%	11.98%	0.76%
Total in File	1,524,716	19.81%	61.65%	81.46%	15.96%	2.59%
Total in Groups	507,067	10.02%	60.53%	70.55%	24.04%	5.41%

NOTES:
Claim lines with invalid provider numbers have been removed from the physician file for all tables.
Carrier file data only.
Outliers above 99 percent have been removed.
Outlier threshold is calculated for each group and in total, therefore, the "Total in File" and "Total in Groups" will not equate to the sum of the groups.
Only physician providers are included in this analysis. Physician provider designation is based on HCFA specialty code.

TABLE D-19 Evaluation and Management Claims Excluding Place of Service 21—Proportion of Beneficiaries Associated with a Percent of Physician Provider Payments Allocated to One Provider

Group	Total Beneficiaries w/ Physician Providers	70–100% of Payments to Provider	50–69% of Payments to Provider	35–49% of Payments to Provider	More than 35% of Payments to Providers	20–34% of Payments to Provider
A—Diabetes, Chronic Heart Failure, & Coronary Artery Disease	32,545	10.99%	20.11%	29.55%	60.66%	33.62%
B—Chronic Heart Failure & Coronary Artery Disease; not Diabetes	44,347	15.12%	22.59%	29.02%	66.73%	29.08%
C—Chronic Heart Failure & Diabetes; not Coronary Artery Disease	19,586	21.96%	25.77%	27.15%	74.88%	22.15%
D—Diabetes & Coronary Artery Disease; not Chronic Heart Failure	52,038	15.63%	24.15%	30.50%	70.28%	26.81%
E—Chronic Heart Failure; not Diabetes & Coronary Artery Disease	43,012	27.08%	26.25%	25.43%	78.76%	18.88%
F—Coronary Artery Disease; not Diabetes & Chronic Heart Failure	137,266	19.42%	25.12%	29.08%	73.62%	23.74%
G—Diabetes; not Chronic Heart Failure & Coronary Artery Disease	179,095	31.21%	28.88%	24.18%	84.27%	13.86%
X—No Condition Category Assigned	1,013,335	35.47%	25.56%	19.80%	80.83%	10.99%
Total in File	1,524,716	31.25%	25.63%	22.24%	79.12%	14.52%
Total in Groups	507,067	23.06%	25.97%	27.18%	76.20%	21.17%

NOTES:
Claim lines with invalid provider numbers have been removed from the physician file for all tables.
Carrier file data only.
Outliers above 99 percent have been removed.
Outlier threshold is calculated for each group and in total, therefore, the "Total in File" and "Total in Groups" will not equate to the sum of the groups.
Only physician providers are included in this analysis. Physician provider designation is based on HCFA specialty code.
The beneficiary is counted once in the highest provider category.

TABLE D-20 Evaluation and Management Claims for Beneficiaries with Hospitalization Excluding Place of Service 21—Proportion of Beneficiaries with 1–10+ Physicians Billing for Care

Group	Total Beneficiaries w/ Physician Providers	1 Physician UPIN per Beneficiary	2-5 Physician UPINs per Beneficiary	Less than 5 Physician UPINs per Beneficiary	6-9 Physician UPINs per Beneficiary	10+ Physician UPINs per Beneficiary
A—Diabetes, Chronic Heart Failure, & Coronary Artery Disease	27,755	2.83%	40.02%	42.85%	38.61%	18.54%
B—Chronic Heart Failure & Coronary Artery Disease; not Diabetes	35,157	4.00%	46.63%	50.64%	35.42%	13.94%
C—Chronic Heart Failure & Diabetes; not Coronary Artery Disease	12,942	5.25%	52.95%	58.20%	31.41%	10.39%
D—Diabetes & Coronary Artery Disease; not Chronic Heart Failure	26,000	3.58%	48.44%	52.02%	35.57%	12.42%
E—Chronic Heart Failure; not Diabetes & Coronary Artery Disease	24,932	7.25%	57.42%	64.68%	28.10%	7.22%
F—Coronary Artery Disease; not Diabetes & Chronic Heart Failure	56,449	4.15%	52.38%	56.53%	34.12%	9.35%
G—Diabetes; not Chronic Heart Failure & Coronary Artery Disease	38,834	5.60%	55.50%	61.10%	30.61%	8.29%
X—No Condition Category Assigned	142,327	6.84%	58.52%	65.35%	27.98%	6.66%
Total in File	364,383	5.45%	53.70%	59.15%	31.41%	9.44%
Total in Groups	221,524	4.57%	50.73%	55.30%	33.69%	11.00%

NOTES:
Claim lines with invalid provider numbers have been removed from the physician file for all tables.
Carrier file data only.
Outliers above 99 percent have been removed.
Outlier threshold is calculated for each group and in total, therefore, the "Total in File" and "Total in Groups" will not equate to the sum of the groups.
Only physician providers are included in this analysis. Physician provider designation is based on HCFA specialty code.

TABLE D-21 Evaluation and Management Claims for Beneficiaries with Hospitalization Excluding Place of Service 21—Proportion of Beneficiaries Associated with a Percent of Physician Provider Payments Allocated to One Provider

Group	Total Beneficiaries w/ Physician Providers	70–100% of Payments to Provider	50–69% of Payments to Provider	35–49% of Payments to Provider	More than 35% of Payments to Providers	20–34% of Payments to Provider
A—Diabetes, Chronic Heart Failure, & Coronary Artery Disease	27,755	9.56%	19.23%	29.35%	58.14%	35.53%
B—Chronic Heart Failure & Coronary Artery Disease; not Diabetes	35,157	12.39%	20.96%	29.33%	62.68%	32.16%
C—Chronic Heart Failure & Diabetes; not Coronary Artery Disease	12,942	16.01%	24.57%	28.78%	69.36%	26.60%
D—Diabetes & Coronary Artery Disease; not Chronic Heart Failure	26,000	10.99%	21.25%	30.43%	62.67%	32.64%
E—Chronic Heart Failure; not Diabetes & Coronary Artery Disease	24,932	19.16%	25.26%	28.26%	72.68%	24.30%
F—Coronary Artery Disease; not Diabetes & Chronic Heart Failure	56,449	12.26%	21.84%	30.69%	64.79%	31.44%
G—Diabetes; not Chronic Heart Failure & Coronary Artery Disease	38,834	15.76%	24.65%	30.46%	70.87%	25.85%
X—No Condition Category Assigned	142,327	17.65%	24.95%	29.15%	71.75%	25.21%
Total in File	364,383	15.06%	23.36%	29.59%	68.01%	28.23%
Total in Groups	221,524	13.43%	22.39%	29.91%	65.73%	30.12%

NOTES:
Claim lines with invalid provider numbers have been removed from the physician file for all tables.
Carrier file data only.
Outliers above 99 percent have been removed.
Outlier threshold is calculated for each group and in total, therefore, the "Total in File" and "Total in Groups" will not equate to the sum of the groups.
Only physician providers are included in this analysis. Physician provider designation is based on HCFA specialty code.
The beneficiary is counted once in the highest provider category.

TABLE D-22 Evaluation and Management Claims for Beneficiaries without Hospitalization Excluding Place of Service 21—Proportion of Beneficiaries with 1–10+ Physicians Billing for Care

Group	Total Beneficiaries w/ Physician Providers	1 Physician UPIN per Beneficiary	2–5 Physician UPINs per Beneficiary	Less than 5 Physician UPINs per Beneficiary	6–9 Physician UPINs per Beneficiary	10+ Physician UPINs per Beneficiary
A—Diabetes, Chronic Heart Failure, & Coronary Artery Disease	4,757	5.91%	59.41%	65.31%	28.61%	6.08%
B—Chronic Heart Failure & Coronary Artery Disease; not Diabetes	9,299	9.51%	64.77%	74.28%	22.45%	3.27%
C—Chronic Heart Failure & Diabetes; not Coronary Artery Disease	6,653	13.53%	66.62%	80.15%	17.81%	2.04%
D—Diabetes & Coronary Artery Disease; not Chronic Heart Failure	26,002	7.13%	65.92%	73.06%	24.27%	2.68%
E—Chronic Heart Failure; not Diabetes & Coronary Artery Disease	18,016	19.10%	65.39%	84.49%	14.70%	0.81%
F—Coronary Artery Disease; not Diabetes & Chronic Heart Failure	80,798	10.54%	67.57%	78.11%	20.00%	1.88%
G—Diabetes; not Chronic Heart Failure & Coronary Artery Disease	140,048	17.71%	69.78%	87.49%	12.51%	
X—No Condition Category Assigned	872,829	27.66%	62.99%	90.65%	9.35%	
Total in File	1,155,308	24.42%	64.43%	88.85%	11.16%	
Total in Groups	285,293	14.26%	68.19%	82.44%	16.57%	0.99%

NOTES:
Claim lines with invalid provider numbers have been removed from the physician file for all tables.
Carrier file data only.
Outliers above 99 percent have been removed.
Outlier threshold is calculated for each group and in total, therefore, the "Total in File" and "Total in Groups" will not equate to the sum of the groups.
Only physician providers are included in this analysis. Physician provider designation is based on HCFA specialty code.

TABLE D-23 Evaluation and Management Claims for Beneficiaries without Hospitalization Excluding Place of Service 21—Proportion of Beneficiaries Associated with a Percent of Physician Provider Payments Allocated to One Provider

Group	Total Beneficiaries w/ Physician Providers	70–100% of Payments to Provider	50–69% of Payments to Provider	35–49% of Payments to Provider	More than 35% of Payments to Providers	20–34% of Payments to Provider
A—Diabetes, Chronic Heart Failure, & Coronary Artery Disease	4,757	19.45%	25.37%	30.84%	75.66%	22.33%
B—Chronic Heart Failure & Coronary Artery Disease; not Diabetes	9,299	25.24%	28.50%	27.56%	81.30%	17.44%
C—Chronic Heart Failure & Diabetes; not Coronary Artery Disease	6,653	33.50%	28.05%	23.73%	85.29%	13.48%
D—Diabetes & Coronary Artery Disease; not Chronic Heart Failure	26,002	20.28%	27.06%	30.57%	77.91%	20.80%
E—Chronic Heart Failure; not Diabetes & Coronary Artery Disease	18,016	38.15%	27.70%	21.52%	87.37%	11.17%
F—Coronary Artery Disease; not Diabetes & Chronic Heart Failure	80,798	24.43%	27.42%	27.95%	79.79%	18.33%
G—Diabetes; not Chronic Heart Failure & Coronary Artery Disease	140,048	35.54%	30.10%	22.41%	88.05%	10.36%
X—No Condition Category Assigned	872,829	38.31%	25.61%	18.25%	82.17%	8.72%
Total in File	1,155,308	36.49%	26.44%	19.93%	82.86%	9.91%
Total in Groups	285,293	30.55%	28.76%	25.03%	84.34%	14.08%

NOTES:
Claim lines with invalid provider numbers have been removed from the physician file for all tables.
Carrier file data only.
Outliers above 99 percent have been removed.
Outlier threshold is calculated for each group and in total, therefore, the "Total in File" and "Total in Groups" will not equate to the sum of the groups.
Only physician providers are included in this analysis. Physician provider designation is based on HCFA specialty code.
The beneficiary is counted once in the highest provider category.

TABLE D-24 Evaluation and Management Claims—Percent of Beneficiaries Seeing Five or Fewer Physicians

	E&M Claims	E&M Claims with Hospitalization	E&M Claims without Hospitalization	E&M Claims: Outpatient Care Only	E&M Claims: Outpatient Care with Hospitalization	E&M Claims: Outpatient Care without Hospitalization
Total in File	75.42%	35.44%	88.09%	81.46%	59.15%	88.85%
Total in Groups	58.79%	29.86%	81.54%	70.55%	55.30%	82.44%

TABLE D-25 Evaluation and Management Claims—Percent of Payments Made to 35 Percent or More Providers

	E&M Claims	E&M Claims with Hospitalization	E&M Claims without Hospitalization	E&M Claims: Outpatient Care only	E&M Claims: Outpatient Care with Hospitalization	E&M Claims: Outpatient Care without Hospitalization
Total in File	76.33%	57.03%	82.38%	79.12%	68.01%	82.86%
Total in Groups	70.48%	53.51%	83.77%	76.20%	65.73%	84.34%

NOTE: Percent of beneficiaries not hospitalized for total in file = 76%; total in groups = 56% (see Table D-16).

E

Pay for Performance in Various Care Settings

Each care setting—dialysis facilities, hospitals, ambulatory physicians, health plans, home health agencies, and skilled nursing facilities—has specific characteristics that need to be considered when planning a pay-for-performance program. This appendix briefly describes each care setting and discusses how rewards could be distributed.

REWARDING DIALYSIS FACILITIES

Background

The treatment of end-stage renal disease (ESRD) is unique in that almost all ESRD patients are covered under Medicare, with only minimal coverage being provided by the private sector or out-of-pocket payment by beneficiaries. Because of the historical placement of dialysis facilities in the Medicare program, however, payment issues are complicated by the fact that payments come from both Part A and Part B. Facility payments (Part A) are capitated, but other, Part B services may be reimbursed in addition to the facility payment. The committee believes that the following three domains should be the focus of initial efforts to provide rewards to dialysis facilities (see Chapter 4):

• *Clinical quality*: Since 1988, a partnership comprising the National Institutes of Health, the Centers for Medicare and Medicaid Services (CMS), and the United States Renal Data System has acted to collect data on this population. (The United States Renal Data System tracks the incidence and prevalence of ESRD and acts to drive the ESRD research agenda.) Five of these measures are currently collected for the Agency for Healthcare Research and Quality's (AHRQ) National Healthcare Quality Report (NHQR). Three of these are outcome measures derived from the University of Michigan. The other two are process measures from the United States Renal Data System. Additionally, the three outcome measures are currently reported on CMS's Dialysis Facility Compare website. Also, as a requirement for payment, all facilities must already be reporting on hematocrit levels as a part of normal reimbursement procedures. The committee believes that dialysis facilities should begin reporting on the measures collected for AHRQ's NHQR (five measures), which could be combined into an equally weighted composite score.

• *Patient-centeredness*: Patients' experiences of care will be measured by a Consumer Assessment of Healthcare Providers and Systems (CAHPS) survey. As of August 2006, an In-Center Hemodialysis (ICH) CAHPS was being finalized to capture the patient's perspective of care in dialysis facilities.

• *Efficiency*: There is a dearth of efficiency measures, and until valid measures are developed, the committee believes that a system should be developed in which dialysis facilities meeting certain thresholds for both clinical quality and patient-centeredness measures are given an additional reward if they are among the most efficient one-third of dialysis facilities. The most efficient third could be calculated using methods for calculating standardized costs for Medicare. For example, Medicare standardized costs over time would be calculated using charges for Medicare Parts A and B (starting at the time of hospitalization and following charges for 90 days) using standard national prices such as an "average" payout per diagnosis-related group or resource-based relative value scale. This would be uniform for all providers and would not include disproportiante share or graduate medical education payments. Using this method, efficiency could be rewarded only when both clinical quality and patient-centered measures were available.

Timing of Pay for Performance

For dialysis facilities, measurement of the three domains is at different levels of development. As the dialysis facilities have been reporting on clinical quality measures as discussed above, the committee believes that rewards could be provided for meeting performance criteria in this domain at the beginning of year 2 (2009). As ICH-CAHPS data were being collected, dialysis facilities would be rewarded for publicly reporting performance data through Dialysis Facility Compare. Beginning in year 3 (2010), as ICH-CAHPS data became available, patient-centeredness would be rewarded based on performance. Efficiency measures could thus begin to be rewarded

TABLE E-1 Dialysis Facility Phasing

	Year 1 (2008)	Year 2 (2009)	Year 3 (2010)
Clinical quality	NHQR measures— pay for public reporting	NHQR measures— pay for performance	NHQR measures— pay for performance
Patient-centeredness		ICH-CAHPS— pay for public reporting	**ICH-CAHPS—pay for performance**
Efficiency			Additional payout to the most efficient 1/3 of facilities meeting thresholds for both clinical quality and patient-centeredness measures

only beginning in year 3. As more measures for each domain were developed, they would be considered for payment based first on public reporting and then on performance. Rewards for public reporting would be smaller than those for performance (see Table E-1).

Example of Pay for Performance for Dialysis Facilities

Measurement of the performance of dialysis facilities and physicians treating ESRD would be based on clinical quality, patient-centeredness, and efficiency. The clinical quality measures would include the following:

Outcomes/Process Measures Table

Outcome Measures	Process Measures
% of hemodialysis patients with urea reduction ratio of 65 or greater	% of dialysis patients registered on a waiting list for transplantation
% of patients with hematocrit of 33 or greater	% of patients with treated chronic kidney failure who receive a transplant within 3 years of renal failure
Patient survival rate	

- *Quality:* A composite score for treatment of ESRD would be assessed to determine whether patients received all the care they should have received. Each measure could be equally weighted, and a straight average could be taken for all five measures.
- *Resource use:* To capture resource use, the committee chose to use longitudinal measures (risk-adjusted mortality) and resource use (standard-

ized costs for Medicare Parts A and B) for all patients at a given dialysis facility.

- *Eligibility for rewards:* The dialysis facility and physicians who billed above a threshold number of evaluation and management (E&M) claims during the subsequent year would be eligible.
- *How to distribute rewards:* There are two choices: (1) rewards could go to dialysis facilities for distribution; or (2) rewards could be split between dialysis facilities (X percent) and physicians (100–X percent), with physician rewards being distributed in proportion to the share of E&M claims.

REWARDING HOSPITALS

Background

Hospitals participating in Medicare are reimbursed by both Medicare Parts A and B. Part A covers facility use, while Part B covers physician payments. Since the adoption of the Medicare Prescription Drug, Improvement, and Modernization Act of 2003 (Public Law 108-173), approximately 4,200 U.S. hospitals have been reporting data on a set of measures agreed upon by the Hospital Quality Alliance (HQA) (hospitalcompare.hhs.gov).

- *Clinical quality:* Previously, hospitals had to report on a set of 10 measures to receive 0.4 percent of their Medicare reimbursement. Now, hospitals are reporting on a set of 20 measures. As these are widely endorsed measures (face validity and relatively strong evidence base), the committee believes that the most recent version of the HQA measure set should be the basis for rewards. These measures should then be combined into a composite for each condition; the composite could be calculated as a sum of the scores of each measure for the given condition. These measures would cut across settings when applicable (see the example for acute myocardial infarction [AMI] in the section below on ambulatory physician care).
- *Patient-centeredness:* Currently the best measures of patients' perspectives on the care they receive derive from the Hospital CAHPS survey. The Hospital CAHPS survey instrument was recently validated and approved for use by CMS. Hospitals have not consistently been collecting and reporting the results of this survey; training will be completed and results will begin to be collected by 2007.
- *Efficiency:* See the above section on dialysis facility care for one possible method.

Timing of Pay for Performance

For hospitals, measurement of the three domains is at different levels of development. As the majority of hospitals have been reporting on clinical

TABLE E-2   Hospital Phasing

	Year 1	Year 2	Year 3
Clinical quality	Hospital Quality Alliance measures— **pay for public reporting**	Hospital Quality Alliance measures— **pay for performance**	Hospital Quality Alliance measures— **pay for performance**
Patient-centeredness	Hospital CAHPS— **pay for public reporting**	Hospital CAHPS— **pay for performance**	Hospital CAHPS— **pay for performance**
Efficiency		Additional payout to the most efficient 1/3 of hospitals meeting thresholds for both clinical quality and patient-centeredness measures	Additional payout to the most efficient 1/3 of hospitals meeting thresholds for both clinical quality and patient-centeredness measures

quality measures as discussed above, the committee believes rewards could be provided for meeting performance criteria for these measures beginning in year 2 (2009). As Hospital CAHPS would just have gotten off the ground, hospitals could be rewarded for publicly reporting these data through Hospital Compare. Beginning in year 2, patient-centeredness could be rewarded based on performance. Efficiency measures could thus begin to be rewarded only beginning in year 2. As more measures for each dimension were developed, they could be considered for payment based first on public reporting and then on performance. Rewards for public reporting would be smaller than those for performance (see Table E-2).

Example of Hospital Pay for Performance

See the example of AMI at the end of the section on ambulatory physicians below.

REWARDING AMBULATORY CARE

Background

Efforts to hold individual physicians accountable for the care they provide are in their early stages because of the basic difficulties involved and the fact that such efforts have never been undertaken on a large scale. There have, however, been some successful smaller-scale examples. An important step toward being able to attribute care in ambulatory settings is a collaborative initiative launched in January 2006 by CMS—the Physician Voluntary Reporting Program. No portion of physician reimbursements has been linked to this initiative (physicians are paid out of Medicare Part B).

- *Clinical quality*: The committee believes that physicians should begin reporting on the measures proposed for the starter set of Ambulatory care Quality Alliance (AQA) measures (currently consisting of 26 measures). Over time, as reporting became more widespread, these measures could be aligned with those used in the Physician Voluntary Reporting Program (currently consisting of 36 measures) as appropriate. Composite scores should be created for each condition.
- *Patient-centeredness*: Patients' experiences of care are currently measured by the CAHPS survey. A survey specifically targeting patients seen at the individual clinician level as part of the Ambulatory CAHPS survey was expected to be released by end of 2006.
- *Efficiency*: See the earlier discussion of dialysis facilities for one possible method.

Timing of Pay for Performance

Reporting on quality measures is not widespread at the level of the individual physician as the basic infrastructure needed to collect and report these data has not yet been broadly adopted at this level. Therefore, the committee proposes the following timeline for implementation.

The first part of year 1 (2008) would likely be spent finalizing performance measures for clinical quality and collecting data, with data cleanup and validation in the latter part of the year. In year 2 (2009), performance reports would be distributed to physicians, and feedback could be provided to reporting physicians, which would be followed by paying for public reporting. In year 3, physicians would be rewarded based on their level of performance. Patient-centered measures for physicians would not be ready for widespread use until 2007; data would have to be collected in the beginning of year 1, and therefore payment for performance based on the results of these patient experience surveys would begin in year 3. Efficiency would be rewarded on for the top one-third of physicians in the nation meeting thresholds for both clinical quality and patient-centeredness. Additional measures would follow the same timeline for implementation as soon as they had been deemed valid (see Table E-3).

Example for Acute Myocardial Infarction

One example of an episode of care that could be paid for according to performance in year 1 is AMI. Measurement of the performance of the

TABLE E-3 Ambulatory Phasing

	Year 1 (2008)	Year 2 (2009)	Year 3 (2010)
Clinical quality		Data back to providers/ feedback period and Ambulatory care Quality Alliance measures— **pay for public reporting**	Ambulatory care Quality Alliance measures— **pay for performance**
Patient-centeredness		Ambulatory CAHPS— **Pay for public reporting**	Ambulatory CAHPS— **pay for performance**
Efficiency			Additional payout to the most efficient 1/3 of physicians meeting thresholds for both clinical quality and patient-centeredness measures

physicians treating such patients would be based on clinical quality, patient-centeredness, and efficiency. The clinical quality measures would include the following:

Acute Myocardial Infarction Measures

Hospital Quality Alliance	Ambulatory care Quality Alliance
Aspirin at arrival for acute myocardial infarction (AMI)	Drug therapy for lowering LDL cholesterol
Aspirin prescribed at discharge for AMI	Beta-blocker treatment after heart attack
Beta-blocker at arrival for AMI	Beta-blocker treatment post–myocardial infarction
Beta-blocker prescribed at discharge for AMI	
AMI inpatient mortality	
Angiotensin-converting enzyme (ACE) inhibitor for left ventricular systolic dysfunction (LVSD)	
Percutaneous coronary intervention (PCI) within 120 minutes of arrival for AMI	
Thrombolytic agent within 30 minutes of arrival for AMI	

Acute Myocardial Infarction Measures

   • *Quality:* A composite score for AMI in each care setting could be formulated to determine whether patients had received all the care they should have received. Each measure could be equally weighted, and a straight average could be taken—one for HQA measures and one for AQA measures.

   • *Resource use:* To capture resource use, the committee proposes longitudinal measures (risk-adjusted mortality) and resource use (standardized costs for Medicare Parts A and B) for all patients at a given hospital with AMI.

   • *Eligibility for rewards:* The hospital and all physicians who billed above a minimum threshold number of E&M claims for the hospital's AMI patients during the subsequent year would be eligible.

   • *How to distribute:* There are two choices: (1) rewards could go to hospitals for distribution; or (2) rewards could be split between hospitals (X percent) and physicians (100–X percent), with physician rewards being distributed in proportion to the share of E&M claims.

REWARDING HEALTH PLAN CARE

Background

   Health plans have been reporting data for more than 10 years through the National Committee for Quality Assurance's (NCQA) Health Plan Employer Data and Information Set (HEDIS). HEDIS, first released by the HMO Group in 1991 and revised by NCQA in 1993, measures the performance of health plans on member satisfaction and delivery of chronic and preventive care for the purpose of accreditation and certification. HEDIS is used by over 90 percent of managed care organizations in the United States. A subset of health plans that work with Medicare, called Medicare Advantage plans, are paid out of Medicare Part C.

   • *Clinical quality:* HEDIS measures are updated annually and are widely endorsed and used. They reflect the following aspects of care: effectiveness of care (preventive screenings; immunizations; treatment of heart attacks, depression, asthma), access/availability of care (access to primary health care and dentistry, timeliness of claims), satisfaction with the experience of care (surveys for adult and child care), health plan stability, use of service, cost of care, informed health care choices, and health plan descriptive information. These data are reported publicly as the quality data within Medicare's Personal Plan Finder, a website dedicated to comparing Medicare health plans.

TABLE E-4 Health Plan Phasing

	Year 1	Year 2	Year 3
Clinical quality	HEDIS measures—**pay for public reporting**	HEDIS measures—**pay for performance**	HEDIS measures—**pay for performance**
Patient-centeredness	CAHPS Health Plan Survey—**pay for public reporting**	CAHPS Health Plan Survey—**pay for performance**	CAHPS Health Plan Survey—**pay for performance**
Efficiency	Additional payout to the most efficient 1/3 of health plans meeting thresholds for both clinical quality and patient-centeredness measures	Additional payout to the most efficient 1/3 of health plans meeting thresholds for both clinical quality and patient-centeredness measures	Additional payout to the most efficient 1/3 of health plans meeting thresholds for both clinical quality and patient-centeredness measures

• *Patient-centeredness*: Health plans have been collecting patient-satisfaction data for years through use of the original CAHPS survey. A more specific survey, the CAHPS health plan survey, is part of the group of Ambulatory CAHPS surveys. It can be used to determine patients' experiences of care provided by their health plan and will be ready for use in 2007.

• *Efficiency*: A system should be developed to supplement the current lack of efficiency measures. See the example for rewarding efficiency in the section on dialysis facilities.

Timing of Pay for Performance

Health plans are very experienced at reporting quality and patient experience data; many have also already begun to provide incentives to their physicians based on performance. Pay for performance could, therefore, be implemented in health plans now. Pay-for-performance programs should include the most up-to-date measures of performance; new measures should be rewarded as they are introduced (see Table E-4).

REWARDING HOME HEALTH CARE

Background

Home health agencies have been able to attribute care to individual facilities, as illustrated by the fact that they have been publicly reporting performance data through CMS since 2003. Federal support for home health care is provided through Medicare, paid out of Part A.

- *Clinical quality*: Home health care has been measured largely through use of the Outcome and Assessment Instrument Set (OASIS). OASIS, implemented in 2000, measures both short- and long-term care in home health agencies. These measures are publicly reported on the Medicare Home Health Compare website.
- *Patient-centeredness*: There currently are no patient-centeredness measures designed specifically for home health care. Efforts to assess patient experiences of care should use the original CAHPS measures, which have long been in use and have widespread support.
- *Efficiency*: See the section on dialysis facilities for one possible method.

Timing of Pay for Performance

As measures of clinical quality are available now, pay for performance on those specific measures could begin in year 1 (2008). CAHPS measures from the original surveys for health plans would be used to characterize patient experiences until a more specific set was available. Because both clinical quality and patient-centeredness measures are available now, efficiency could also be assessed (see Table E-5).

TABLE E-5 Home Health Care Phasing

	Year 1 (2008)	Year 2 (2009)	Year 3 (2010)
Clinical quality	OASIS measures— **pay for performance**	OASIS measures— **pay for performance**	OASIS measures— **pay for performance**
Patient-centeredness	CAHPS measures— **pay for performance**	CAHPS measures— **pay for performance**	CAHPS measures— **pay for performance**
Efficiency	Additional payout to the most efficient 1/3 of home health agencies meeting thresholds for both clinical quality and patient-centeredness measures	Additional payout to the most efficient 1/3 of home health agencies meeting thresholds for both clinical quality and patient-centeredness measures	Additional payout to the most efficient 1/3 of home health agencies meeting thresholds for both clinical quality and patient-centeredness measures

Example of Pay for Performance for Home Health Care

Measurement of the performance of the physicians treating home health care patients would be based on clinical quality, patient-centeredness, and efficiency. The clinical quality measures would include the following:

- *Quality:* A composite score for home health care in each care setting would be formulated to determine whether patients had received all the care they should have received. Each measure would be equally weighted, and a straight average would be taken.
- *Resource use:* To capture resource use, the committee proposes standardized costs for Medicare Part A for all patients at a given home health agency.
- *Eligibility for rewards:* Home health agencies that billed above a minimum threshold number of claims for patients during the subsequent year would be eligible.
- *How to distribute:* Rewards would be distributed to the home health agencies based on performance.

OASIS Measures	
1. Improvement in ambulation/ locomotion	Patients who get better at walking or moving around in a wheelchair safely
2. Improvement in transferring	Patients who get better at getting in and out of bed
3. Improvement in toileting	Patients who get better at getting to and from the toilet
4. Improvement in pain interfering with activity	Patients who have less pain when moving around
5. Improvement in bathing	Patients who get better at bathing
6. Improvement in management of oral medications	Patients who get better at taking their medications correctly (by mouth)
7. Improvement in upper body dressing	Patients who get better at getting dressed
8. Stabilization in bathing	Patients who stay the same (don't get worse) at bathing
9. Acute care hospitalization	Percentage of patients who had to be admitted to the hospital
10. Emergent care	Percentage of patients who need urgent, unplanned medical care
11. Improvement in confusion frequency	Patients who are confused less often

REWARDING SKILLED NURSING FACILITY CARE

Background

The majority of nursing home care is paid for by Medicaid and private payers. Medicare pays for a specific type of nursing home care, called skilled nursing care, through Medicare Part A. This care constitutes 25 percent of all nursing home care.

- *Clinical quality:* The Minimum Data Set evaluates care in nursing homes. There are only three measures in this set that pertain to skilled nursing facilities. Evaluation of nursing homes is available through the Medicare Nursing Home Compare website.
- *Patient-centeredness:* A Nursing Home CAHPS survey is still being developed to assess both patient and family experiences of care. Field testing was completed in January 2006; the final approval date for the instrument has yet to be determined.
- *Efficiency:* See the section on hospital care for one possible method.

Timing of Pay for Performance

As described in Chapter 5, measures are not yet available that can adequately characterize care provided by skilled nursing facilities. Until such measures are developed, pay for performance should not be implemented in this setting. Once the necessary measures were available, implementation would proceed in a fashion similar to that for the other settings where pay for public reporting would precede pay for performance.

F

Acronym List

ABIM	American Board of Internal Medicine
ABMS	American Board of Medical Specialties
ACC	American College of Cardiology
ACHP	Alliance of Community Health Plans
ACP	American College of Physicians
AMA	American Medical Association
AHRQ	Agency for Healthcare Research and Quality
AQA	Ambulatory care Quality Alliance
BIPA	Benefits Improvement and Protection Act
CAHPS	Consumer Assessment of Healthcare Providers and Systems
CHI	Consolidated Health Informatics
CMS	Centers for Medicare and Medicaid Services
DHHS	Department of Health and Human Services
DRG	diagnosis-related group
EHR	electronic health record
ESRD	end-stage renal disease
GAO	Government Accountability Office
GDP	gross domestic product
GP	general practitioner

HEDIS	Health Plan Employer Data and Information Set
HIPAA	Health Insurance Portability and Accountability Act
HMO	health maintenance organization
HQA	Hospital Quality Alliance
IHA	Integrated Healthcare Association
IOM	Institute of Medicine
MedPAC	Medicare Payment Advisory Commission
NCQA	National Committee for Quality Assurance
NHIN	National Health Information Network
NHS	National Health Service
NQCB	National Quality Coordination Board
PDCA (PDSA)	Plan-Do-Check/Study-Act
PPO	preferred provider organization
RHIO	Regional Health Information Organization
RBRVS	resource-based relative value scale
RFR	reduction in failure rate
SCHIP	State Children's Health Insurance Program
SGR	sustainable growth rate
SNF	skilled nursing facility
STS	Society of Thoracic Surgeons
USRDS	United States Renal Data System

G

Biographies

AUTHORING COMMITTEE

Steven A. Schroeder, M.D., *Chair,* is distinguished professor of health and health care, Division of General Internal Medicine, Department of Medicine, University of California, San Francisco (UCSF), where he also heads the Smoking Cessation Leadership Center. The Center, funded by The Robert Wood Johnson Foundation, works with leaders of American health professional organizations and health care institutions to increase the rate at which patients who smoke are offered help to quit. Between 1990 and 2002 he was president and chief executive officer (CEO) of The Robert Wood Johnson Foundation. During his term of office the foundation made grant expenditures of almost $4 billion in pursuit of its mission of improving the health and health care of the American people. During those 12$\frac{1}{2}$ years the foundation developed new programs in substance abuse prevention and treatment, care at the end of life, and health insurance expansion for children, among others. In 1999, it reorganized into health and health care groups, reflecting the twin components of its mission. Dr. Schroeder graduated from Stanford University and Harvard Medical School, and trained in internal medicine at the Harvard Medical Service of Boston City Hospital and in epidemiology as an Epidemic Intelligence Service Officer of the Centers for Disease Control and Prevention. He held faculty appointments at Harvard, George Washington, and UCSF. At both George Washington and UCSF he was founding medical director of a university- sponsored health maintenance organization (HMO), and at UCSF he founded the

222

company's division of general internal medicine. Dr. Schroeder has produced more than 260 publications in the fields of clinical medicine, health care financing and organization, prevention, public health, and the workforce. He recently completed his term as chair of the American Legacy Foundation and chair of the International Review Committee of the Ben Gurion School of Medicine. He is a member of the editorial board of the *New England Journal of Medicine* and the Harvard Overseers, and a director of the James Irvine Foundation, the Save Ellis Island Foundation, and the Charles R. Drew University of Medicine and Science. He holds six honorary doctoral degrees and has received numerous awards.

Robert D. Reischauer, Ph.D., *Co-Chair, Pay for Performance Subcommittee,** is president of the Urban Institute, a nonprofit, nonpartisan policy research and education organization that examines the social, economic, and governance problems facing the nation. He served as director of the Congressional Budget Office (CBO) between 1989 and 1995 and was CBO's assistant director for human resources and deputy director during 1977 to 1981. Dr. Reischauer has been a senior fellow in the Economic Studies Program of the Brookings Institution (1986–1989 and 1995–2000) and senior vice president of the Urban Institute (1981–1986). He is an economist with an undergraduate degree from Harvard and a Ph.D. in economics and masters in international affairs from Columbia University. Dr. Reischauer is a member of the Harvard Corporation and serves on the boards of several educational and nonprofit organizations. He is vice-chair of the Medicare Payment Advisory Commission (MedPAC) and served as chair of the National Academy of Social Insurance's project "Restructuring Medicare for the Long Term" from 1995 through 2004.

Gail R. Wilensky, Ph.D., *Co-Chair, Pay for Performance Subcommittee,** is a senior fellow at Project HOPE, an international health education foundation, where she analyzes and develops policies relating to health reform and to ongoing changes in the medical marketplace. Dr. Wilensky testifies frequently before congressional committees; acts as an advisor to members of Congress and other elected officials; and speaks nationally and internationally before professional, business, and consumer groups. From 2001 to 2003, she cochaired the President's Task Force to Improve Health Care Delivery for Our Nation's Veterans, which addressed health care for both veterans and military retirees. From 1997 to 2001 she chaired the Medicare Payment Advisory Commission, which advises Congress on payment and other issues relating to Medicare, and from 1995 to 1997 she chaired the

---

*Member of the Subcommittee on Pay for Performance.

Physician Payment Review Commission. Previously, she served as deputy assistant to President G.H.W. Bush for policy development, advising him on health and welfare issues. Prior to that, she was administrator of the Healthcare Financing Administration (HCFA), overseeing the Medicare and Medicaid programs. Dr. Wilensky is an elected member of the Institute of Medicine (IOM) and its Governing Council, serves as a trustee of the Combined Benefits Fund of the United Mineworkers of America and the American Heart Association, and is on the Advisory Board of the National Institute of Health Care Management. She is an advisor to The Robert Wood Johnson Foundation and The Commonwealth Fund, immediate past chair of the Board of Directors of AcademyHealth, and a director on several corporate boards. Dr. Wilensky received a bachelor's degree in psychology and a Ph.D. in economics at the University of Michigan.

Bobbie Berkowitz, Ph.D., R.N., F.A.A.N., is alumni endowed professor of nursing at the University of Washington (UW) School of Nursing and adjunct professor in the School of Public Health and Community Medicine. She directs the "Turning Point" initiative funded by The Robert Wood Johnson Foundation and the Center for the Advancement of Health Disparities Research funded by the National Institute of Nursing Research. She serves on the board of directors as vice-chair of Qualis Health, the Quality Improvement Organization of Washington State. Before joining UW, Dr. Berkowitz was deputy secretary of health for the Washington State Department of Health. She is a member of the board of trustees for Group Health Cooperative, a fellow in the American Academy of Nursing, and a member of the IOM. She served as co-chair of the IOM Committee on Using Performance Monitoring to Improve Community Health and as vice-chair of the IOM/Transportation Research Board Committee on Physical Activity, Health, Transportation, and Land Use. She holds a Ph.D. in nursing science from Case Western Reserve University.

Donald M. Berwick, M.D., M.P.P., is president and CEO of the Institute for Healthcare Improvement (IHI), a not-for-profit organization helping to accelerate the improvement of health care throughout the world. He is clinical professor of pediatrics and health care policy at Harvard Medical School and professor of health policy and management at Harvard School of Public Health. He is also a pediatrician, an associate in pediatrics at Boston's Children's Hospital, and a consultant in pediatrics at Massachusetts General Hospital. Dr. Berwick has published over 110 scientific articles in numerous professional journals on subjects relating to health care policy, decision analysis, technology assessment, and health care quality management. He serves on the IOM's Governing Council and the IOM's Board on Global Health. He is also a member of several editorial boards, including that of the *Journal of the American Medical Association*. A summa cum laude graduate of Harvard College, Dr. Berwick holds a master of public policy degree from the John F. Kennedy School of Government and an M.D. cum laude from Harvard Medical School.

Bruce E. Bradley, M.B.A., is director of Health Care Plan Strategy and Public Policy, Health Care Initiatives, for General Motors Corporation in Pontiac, Michigan. He is responsible for health care–related strategy and public policy, with a focus on quality measurement and improvement, consumer engagement, and cost-effectiveness. General Motors provides health care coverage for over 1.1 million employees, retirees, and their dependents, with an annual expense of $5.2 billion. Mr. Bradley joined General Motors in June 1996 after 5 years as corporate manager of Managed Care for GTE Corporation. In addition to his health care management experience at GTE, he spent nearly 20 years in health plan and HMO management. From 1972 to 1980 he was executive director of the Matthew Thornton Health Plan, Nashua, New Hampshire. From 1980 to 1990 he was president and CEO of the Rhode Island Group Health Association in Providence, a staff model HMO. He was cofounder of the HMO Group (now the Alliance of Community Health Plans), a national corporation of 15 nonprofit, independent group practice HMOs, and the HMO Group Insurance Co., Ltd. Mr. Bradley has gained recognition for his work in achieving health plan quality improvement and for his efforts in developing the Health Plan Employer Data and Information Set measures and processes. He is a board member of the National Quality Forum (NQF), past member of the board of the Foundation for Accountability, board member of the American Board of Internal Medicine Foundation, past board member of the Academy for Health Services Research and Policy, and founding member and past chair of the Leapfrog Group board. A native of Pelham, New York, Mr. Bradley holds a bachelor's degree in psychology from Yale University (1967) and a master's degree in business and health care administration from the Wharton School at the University of Pennsylvania (1972).

Janet M. Corrigan, Ph.D.,* is president and CEO of the NQF, a private, not-for-profit membership organization established in 1999 to develop and implement a national strategy for health care quality measurement and reporting. The NQF portfolio includes the endorsement of performance measurement consensus standards, educational programs for health care leaders on key environmental trends, and award recognition programs. Dr. Corrigan was instrumental in organizing the merger between NQF and the

---

*Member of the Subcommittee on Pay for Performance.

National Committee for Quality Health Care (NCQHC), where she served as president and CEO from June 2005 to March 2006. Prior to joining NCQHC in June 2005, she was senior board director at the IOM, where she was responsible for the Board on Health Care Services' portfolio of initiatives on quality and safety, health services organization and financing, and health insurance issues. She provided leadership for the IOM's *Quality Chasm* series, which includes 10 reports produced during her tenure, among them *To Err Is Human: Building a Safer Health System* and *Crossing the Quality Chasm: A New Health System for the 21st Century.* She serves on the boards of the Baldrige Board of Overseers and the National Center for Healthcare Leadership. She received her doctorate in health services research, a master of industrial engineering degree from the University of Michigan, and master's degrees in business administration and community health from the University of Rochester.

Karen Davis, Ph.D.,* is president of The Commonwealth Fund, a national philanthropy engaged in independent research on health and social issues. A nationally recognized economist, she has had a distinguished career in public policy and research. She served as deputy assistant secretary for health policy in the U.S. Department of Health and Human Services from 1977 to 1980 and holds the distinction of being the first woman to head a U.S. Public Health Service agency. Prior to her government career, Dr. Davis was a senior fellow at the Brookings Institution in Washington, D.C., a visiting scholar at Harvard University, and an assistant professor of economics at Rice University. She was chair of health policy and management at the Johns Hopkins Bloomberg School of Public Health from 1981 to 1992. She also serves on the board of Geisinger Health System. She is the recipient of the 2000 Baxter-Allegiance Foundation Prize for Health Services Research and the 2006 AcademyHealth Distinguished Investigator Award. She is a former president of AcademyHealth. Dr. Davis received her doctorate in economics from Rice University and was awarded an honorary doctorate in humane letters from The Johns Hopkins University in 2001.

Nancy-Ann Min DeParle, J.D., is a senior advisor to JPMorgan Partners, LLC, and adjunct professor of health care systems at the Wharton School of the University of Pennsylvania. From 1997 to 2000, she served as administrator of HCFA, now the Centers for Medicare and Medicaid Services. Before joining HCFA, Ms. DeParle was associate director for health and personnel at the White House Office of Management and Budget. From 1987 to 1989 she served as the Tennessee commissioner of human services. She is

---

*Member of the Subcommittee on Pay for Performance.

a member of MedPAC; a trustee of The Robert Wood Johnson Foundation; and a board member of Cerner Corporation, DaVita, Boston Scientific, Triad Hospitals, and the NQF. Ms. DeParle received a bachelor's degree from the University of Tennessee; bachelor's and master's degrees from Oxford University, where she was a Rhodes Scholar; and a J.D. degree from Harvard Law School.

Elliott S. Fisher, M.D., M.P.H.,* is professor of medicine and community and family medicine and director of the Institute for the Evaluation of Medical Practice at the Center for the Evaluative Clinical Sciences, Hanover, New Hampshire, and senior associate of the VA Outcomes Group, Veterans Administration Medical Center, White River Junction, Vermont. He is a general internist and former Robert Wood Johnson clinical scholar with broad expertise in the use of administrative databases and survey research methods in health systems evaluation. His research has focused on exploring the causes and consequences of variations in clinical practice and health care spending across U.S. regions and among health care providers.

Richard G. Frank, Ph.D., is Margaret T. Morris professor of health economics in the Department of Health Care Policy at Harvard Medical School. He is also a research associate with the National Bureau of Economic Research. Dr. Frank is a member of the IOM. He advises several state mental health and substance abuse agencies on issues related to managed care and financing of care. He also serves as coeditor for the *Journal of Health Economics.* Dr. Frank was awarded the Georgescu-Roegen prize from the Southern Economic Association for his collaborative work on drug pricing, the Carl A. Taube Award from the American Public Health Association for outstanding contributions to mental health services and economics research, and the Emily Mumford Medal from Columbia University's Department of Psychiatry. In 2002 Dr. Frank received the John Eisenberg Mentorship Award from National Research Service Awards.

Robert S. Galvin, M.D.,* is director of Global Health Care for General Electric (GE). He is in charge of the design and performance of GE's health programs, totaling over $3 billion annually, and oversees the 1 million patient encounters that take place in GE's 220 medical clinics in more than 25 countries. Drawing on his clinical expertise and training in Six Sigma, Dr. Galvin has been an advocate and leader in extending the benefits of this methodology to health care. He has focused on issues of market-based health policy and financing, with special interests in measurement transpar-

---

*Member of the Subcommittee on Pay for Performance.

ency, payment system reform, and the assessment and coverage of new technologies. He is a past member of the Strategic Framework Board of the NQF and is currently on the board of the National Committee for Quality Assurance. He is a cofounder of the Leapfrog Group, the founder of Bridges to Excellence, and a member of the Advisory Group of the Council on Health Care Economics and Policy. Dr. Galvin is widely published on issues affecting the purchaser side of health care. He is professor adjunct of medicine at Yale, where he directs the seminar series on the private sector for the Robert Wood Johnson Clinical Scholars fellowship. He is a fellow of the American College of Physicians.

David H. Gustafson, Ph.D., is a research professor at the University of Wisconsin, Madison, where he directs the Center of Excellence in Cancer Communications (designated by the National Cancer Institute) and the Network for the Improvement of Addiction Treatment (supported by The Robert Wood Johnson Foundation and the federal government's Center for Substance Abuse Treatment). His research focuses on the use of systems engineering methods and models in individual and organizational change. Much of his research centers on the development and evaluation of health systems to support people facing serious health problems such as cancer. His randomized controlled trials and field tests have helped in understanding the acceptance, use, and impact of e-health on quality of life, behavior change, and health service utilization. His research has also contributed to organizational improvement, with particular attention to models that predict and explain organizational change. Dr. Gustafson is a fellow of the Association for Health Services Research and of the American Medical Informatics Association and a fellow and past vice-chair of the board of IHI. He also chaired the recent Federal Science Panel on Interactive Communications in Health and is chair of the Health Institute. He is a former member of the University of Wisconsin Athletic Board.

Mary Anne Koda-Kimble, Pharm.D., is dean of the School of Pharmacy at UCSF, where she teaches and has cared for patients at the UCSF Diabetes Center. She holds the Thomas J. Long Endowed Professorship and previously served as chair of the Department of Clinical Pharmacy. Dr. Koda-Kimble received her Pharm.D. from UCSF and joined its faculty in 1970, where she was involved in developing an innovative clinical pharmacy curriculum. She is a member of the United States Pharmacopoeia board of trustees and was vice-chair of the Accreditation Council of Pharmaceutical Education board of Directors. She is past president of the American Association of Colleges of Pharmacy and has served on the California State Board of Pharmacy, the Food and Drug Administration's Nonprescription

Drugs Advisory Committee, and many other boards and task forces of national professional associations. Dr. Koda-Kimble is frequently invited to address national and international groups and has produced many publications, the best known of which is *Applied Therapeutics*, a text widely used by health professional students and practitioners throughout the world.

Alan R. Nelson, M.D., is an internist–endocrinologist who was in private practice in Salt Lake City, Utah, until becoming CEO of the American Society of Internal Medicine (ASIM) in 1992. Following the merger of ASIM with the American College of Physicians (ACP) in 1998, Dr. Nelson headed the Washington Office of ACP–ASIM until his semiretirement in January 2000; he currently serves as special advisor to the executive vice president/ CEO of the college. He was president of the American Medical Association and from 2000 to 2006 served as a member of MedPAC, which advises Congress on Medicare issues. A member of the IOM, he was chair of the IOM Committee on Ethnic and Racial Disparities in Health Care and is a coeditor of the study report, *Unequal Treatment: Confronting Racial and Ethnic Disparities in Health Care*. Dr. Nelson attended Utah State University and received his M.D. from Northwestern University in 1958.

Norman C. Payson, M.D., was selected to be chairman of the board of Concentra, Inc. As chairman, he oversees its strategic direction, management development and guidance, and governance. Dr. Payson was previously CEO of two publicly traded health plans—Oxford Health Plans as the "turnaround CEO" (1998–2002) and Healthsource, Inc. as cofounder and CEO (1985– 1997). Prior to joining Healthsource, Dr. Payson was CEO and Medical Director of a 120-doctor physician group practice. Dr. Payson is a board member of the Mailman School of Public Health at Columbia University; Medicine in Need Corporation, a charitable biotechnology company; and the City of Hope in Los Angeles. He serves on the advisory board of the Health Sciences Technology Division at MIT–Harvard Medical School and the board of overseers at Dartmouth Medical School. Dr. Payson is a graduate of the Massachusetts Institute of Technology and Dartmouth Medical School. He lives in Hopkinton, New Hampshire, with his wife, Melinda.

William A. Peck, M.D., became Alan A. and Edith L. Wolff Distinguished Professor of Medicine and director of the Washington University Center for Health Policy in 2003. From 1989 to 2003 he served as dean of Washington University School of Medicine and vice chancellor for medical affairs (executive vice chancellor from 1993 to 2003), and president of the Washington University Medical Center. Dr. Peck was awarded an honorary doctor of science degree from the University of Rochester in 2000. His academic activities include original investigations in bone and mineral metabolism, extensive clinical teaching, as well as patient care experience. He was founding president of the National Osteoporosis Foundation and has served on the editorial boards of multiple journals, on numerous national and international medical and scientific panels, and on advisory boards of major pharmaceutical companies. He has held numerous lectureships and society memberships, including the American Society for Clinical Investigation, the Association of American Physicians, and the Institute of Medicine (NAS). Dr. Peck is the recipient of many international, national, and regional awards. He serves on the boards of Allied Health Care Products, Angelica Corporation, TIAA-CREF Trust Company, and Research!America (vice-chair), and is a trustee of the University of Rochester. Dr. Peck is past chairman of the American Association of Medical Colleges. He has been a consultant for many major pharmaceutical companies.

Neil R. Powe, M.D., M.P.H., M.B.A.,* is professor of medicine, professor of health policy and management, and professor of epidemiology at the Johns Hopkins University School of Medicine and the Johns Hopkins Bloomberg School of Public Health. He also is director of the Welch Center for Prevention, Epidemiology and Clinical Research, an interdisciplinary research and training center at the Johns Hopkins Medical Institutions focused on population-based and health services research. Dr. Powe's research has involved clinical epidemiology, technology assessment, patient outcomes research, and health services research in many areas of medicine. He has also studied physician decision making and other determinants of the use of medical practices, including payers' decisions about insurance coverage for new medical technologies; the effect of financial incentives on the use of technology; efficiency and outcomes in for-profit versus nonprofit health care institutions; and the relationships among hospital volume, technology, and outcomes. He has extensive experience in developing and measuring outcomes and quality of care for chronic kidney disease and is author of more than 250 articles. Dr. Powe received his M.D. from Harvard Medical School, M.P.H. from Harvard School of Public Health, and M.B.A. from the University of Pennsylvania. He completed his residency at the Hospital of the University of Pennsylvania, where he was also a Robert Wood Johnson Clinical Scholar and fellow in the Division of General Internal Medicine. Dr. Powe is a member of the American Society of Clinical Investigation, the Association of American Physicians, and the American Society of Epidemiology.

---

*Member of the Subcommittee on Pay for Performance.

Christopher Queram, M.A.,* has been president/CEO of the Wisconsin Collaborative for Healthcare Quality (WCHQ) since November 2005. The collaborative is a nonprofit, 501c3 voluntary consortium of organizations leading and working together to improve the quality and cost-effectiveness of health care for the people of Wisconsin. The collaborative develops and reports comparative measures of health care performance; designs and promotes quality improvement initiatives; and advocates for enlightened policy to support its work. Prior to joining WCHQ, Mr. Queram served as CEO of the Employer Health Care Alliance Cooperative (the Alliance) of Madison, Wisconsin, a health care purchasing cooperative owned by more than 160 member companies. In addition to his responsibilities at WCHQ, Mr. Queram is a board member of the Joint Commission on Accreditation of Health Care Organizations and Delta Dental of Wisconsin, a member of the "Principals" for the Hospital Quality Alliance (HQA), and a member of the steering committee for the Wisconsin Hospital Association's CheckPoint quality reporting initiative. Previously, he served as board member of the Leapfrog Group and the NQF, as well as a member of the IOM's Committee on the Consequences of Uninsurance and President Clinton's Advisory Commission on Consumer Protection and Quality in the Health Care Industry. Mr. Queram holds a master of arts degree in health services administration from the University of Wisconsin, Madison, and is a fellow in the American College of Healthcare Executives.

William C. Richardson, Ph.D., is past president and CEO emeritus of the W. K. Kellogg Foundation and president emeritus of The Johns Hopkins University. Before joining the foundation in August 1995, Dr. Richardson was president of Johns Hopkins, a position he had held since 1990, and professor of health policy and management at the university. Dr. Richardson has been a member of the IOM since 1981, a fellow of the American Academy of Arts and Sciences, and a member of the American Public Health Association. He has chaired several IOM committees. He has also served on the boards of the Council of Michigan Foundations and the Council on Foundations (trustee and chair). He serves as well on the board of directors of the Kellogg Company, CSX Corporation, the Bank of New York, and Exelon Corporation. Dr. Richardson is a graduate of Trinity College and the University of Chicago.

Cheryl M. Scott, M.H.A.,* is currently president emerita for Group Health Cooperative (GHC), one of the the nation's largest consumer-governed, nonprofit health care systems. From 1997 to 2004, she was GHC's president and

---

*Member of the Subcommittee on Pay for Performance.

CEO. Prior to assuming her position in 1997, she served as GHC's executive vice president/chief operating officer. Ms. Scott is a clinical professor in the Department of Health Services at the University of Washington. At the national level, she served on the board of the Alliance of Community Plans (trustee and chair) and the board of America's Health Insurance Plans. She currently serves as board chair for the Health Technology Center and is a trustee for the Washington State Life Sciences Discovery Fund. Ms. Scott received a bachelor's degree in communications and a master's degree in health administration from the University of Washington.

Stephen M. Shortell, Ph.D., M.P.H., is a prominent researcher in health policy and organization behavior at the University of California, Berkeley, and is dean of the School of Public Health. Dr. Shortell is known as a leading academic voice advocating reform of the nation's health system. His research has helped establish determinants of health outcomes and quality of care for health care organizations. As Blue Cross of California distinguished professor of health policy and management, Dr. Shortell holds a joint appointment at UC Berkeley's School of Public Health and the Haas School of Business. He also is affiliated with UC Berkeley's Department of Sociology and UC San Francisco's Institute for Health Policy Studies. Dr. Shortell is an elected member of the IOM. He has received the Baxter-Allegiance Prize, considered the highest honor worldwide in the field of health services research. He also has received the Distinguished Investigator Award from the Association for Health Services Research and the Gold Medal award from the American College of Healthcare Executives for his contributions to the field. He serves on the boards of the Health Research and Educational Trust and the National Center for Healthcare Leadership. Dr. Shortell received his bachelor's degree from the University of Notre Dame; his master's degree in public health from the University of California, Los Angeles; and his Ph.D. in behavioral science from the University of Chicago. Before coming to UC Berkeley in 1998, he held teaching and research positions at Northwestern University, the University of Washington, and the University of Chicago.

Samuel O. Thier, M.D., is professor of medicine and professor of health care policy at Harvard Medical School. He was president and CEO of Partners HealthCare System from 1996 to 2002. From 1994 to 1997 he was president of the Massachusetts General Hospital; he was Brandeis University's president during the previous 3 years. He served 6 years as president of the IOM and 11 years as chair of the Department of Internal Medicine at Yale University School of Medicine, where he was Sterling professor. Dr. Thier is an authority on internal medicine and kidney disease and is also known for his expertise in national health policy, medical education, and biomedical research. Born in New York, he attended Cornell University and received his medical degree from the State University of New York at Syracuse in 1960. He served on the medical staff of Massachusetts General Hospital as an intern, resident, chief resident in medicine, and chief of the renal unit, and held a faculty appointment at Harvard. Prior to joining the faculty of Yale in 1975, he was professor and vice-chair of the Department of Medicine at the University of Pennsylvania. He has received several honorary degrees and the UC Medal of the University of California, San Francisco. He has served as president of the American Federation of Clinical Research and chair of the American Board of Internal Medicine and is a master of the American College of Physicians, a fellow of the American Academy of Arts and Sciences, and a member of the American Philosophical Society. Dr. Thier is a director of Charles River Laboratories, Inc., The Commonwealth Fund (chair), the Federal Reserve Bank of Boston, and Merck & Co., Inc., and a member of the Board of Overseers of TIAA-CREF and the Board of Overseers of Cornell University Medical College.

ADVISORY SUBCOMMITTEE ON PAY FOR PERFORMANCE

The members of the advisory subcommittee listed below supported, but were not part of, the main authoring committee.

Stephanie Alexander, M.B.A., is senior vice president for Premier Healthcare Informatics. She has been active in the health care decision-support business for 20 years and speaks regularly on the importance of measurement to realize consistent health care improvement. Earlier in her career, she served as project manager for operational improvement consulting engagements, resulting in multimillion dollar savings for health systems. She also served as director of process improvement for a 450-bed hospital and managed process improvement programs in several hospitals. She was deeply involved in the development of Premier's *Perspective*™ system, which hospitals use for measurement, benchmarking, and reporting of clinical performance. She is an engineering graduate of North Carolina State University and holds an MBA from the University of North Carolina at Chapel Hill.

Charles D. Baker is president and CEO of Harvard Pilgrim Health Care, Inc. (HPHC), one of New England's leading nonprofit health plans. Harvard Pilgrim and its affiliates are licensed to provide comprehensive health insurance solutions in Massachusetts, Maine, and New Hampshire. Its provider network has more than 22,000 physicians and 135 hospitals in Massachusetts, Maine, New Hampshire, and Rhode Island. HPHC offers health and benefit plan solutions to over 970,000 members in New England. He was brought in as CEO in mid-1999 to turn around the organization's financial performance. HPHC has posted positive gains for 24 consecutive quarters, is rated Ba1 with a "stable" outlook by Moody's Investors Services, and has over $325 million in net worth. In addition, HPHC finished first in the country for two years in a row on the National Committee for Quality Assurance's (NCQA's) annual ranking of health plan performance. HPHC was also featured this year as the #1 health plan in the country in a special issue of U.S. News & World Report, and has won several JD Power "Plan of Distinction" awards. HPHC is a market leader in the development and use of secure, online tools to reduce administrative costs and improve the accuracy and speed of health care transactions. Its chief tool, *HPHConnect*, is serving thousands of employers, providers and members, offering 24/7 administrative support for a wide variety of transactions. *HPHConnect* currently supports over 1 million transactions a month for HPHC providers, employers and members.

Arnold M. Epstein, M.D., M.A., is chairman of the Department of Health Policy and Management at the Harvard University School of Public Health where he is the John H. Foster Professor, and chief of the Section on Health Services and Policy Research in the Department of Medicine at the Brigham and Women's Hospital. Dr. Epstein's research interests focus on quality of care and access to care for disadvantaged populations. Recently his efforts have focused on racial and ethnic disparities in care, public reporting of quality performance data and incentives for quality improvement. He has published 175 articles on these and other topics. His book, *Falling Through the Safety Net, Insurance Status and Access to Health Care*, won the Kulp Wright Award by the American Risk and Insurance Association in 1994 for the best new book on life and health insurance. During 1993–1994, he worked for the White House where he had staff responsibility for policy issues related to the health care delivery system, especially quality management. He was Vice Chair of the IOM Committee on Developing a National Report on Health Care Quality, and Co-Chair of the Performance Measurement Coordinating Committee of the Joint Commission on the Accreditation of Health Care Organizations (JCAHO), the NCQA, and the American Medical Association. He has served as Chairman of the Board of AcademyHealth and remains on its Board now. He serves on JCAHO's Advisory Council on Performance Measurement. He has served on several editorial boards including *Health Services Research* and the *Annals of Internal Medicine*. He has been elected to the American Society for Clinical Investigation and the American Association of Professors. He is currently Associate Editor for Health Policy at the *New England Journal of Medicine* and a member of the IOM.

Sam Ho, M.D., is currently chief medical officer for UnitedHealthcare's Pacific and Southwest regions, and is responsible for the clinical advancement of members in the western United States. Previously, he was the executive vice president and chief medical officer for PacifiCare Health Systems, and was responsible for improving the quality, costs, and access for both commercial and Medicare beneficiaries. He led all quality improvement and clinical management programs, medical informatics, and established innovative programs and results in such areas as provider profiling; consumer transparency; value-based networks and product design; pay for performance; consumer incentives for healthier behavior; disease management; and health IT. Such efforts helped distinguish PacifiCare as a pioneer in the managed care industry, earning awards from the National Business Group on Health, the NCQA, the Foundation for Accountability, and the Disease Management Association of America. In 2003 he received the Health Insurance Association of America's 2003 Innovator Award for innovative leadership in health insurance, and he is nationally recognized in the areas of health policy, program innovation, and operational execution with continuously improved results.

Barbara Manard, Ph.D., a health policy researcher and consultant with over 20 years of experience, joined the American Association of Homes and Services for the Aging (AAHSA) in 2003 as vice president of long-term care/health strategies. Prior to joining AAHSA, she served as vice president of The Lewin Group (1981–1987) and subsequently as president of a Maryland-based research and consulting firm, the Manard Company (1998–2002). In 1998, she served as a Special Expert Consultant to the Office of the Secretary (ASPE), United States Department of Health and Human Services, to assist with technical and policy issues related to implementing post–acute care Medicare payment system changes mandated by Congress. In 2001, she assisted ASPE with a project regarding post–acute care assessment instruments, reference vocabularies, and electronic medical records. Prior to joining the Lewin Group, Dr. Manard served as a policy analyst at ASPE and as an assistant professor of sociology at the University of California (Riverside). She received her doctorate in sociology from the University of Virginia, a certificate in health planning from the University of Virginia School of Medicine, and an AB from Vassar College.

L. Gordon Moore, M.D., a faculty member of the IHI, he works with office practice teams from across the United States, helping them pilot and implement open/advanced access scheduling, office efficiency, and the improvement of chronic illness and preventive care with the McColl Institute's Care Model. He is coleading a clinical transformation project as part of a groundbreaking initiative to re-weave the safety net in Rochester, New York (www.rsafetynetproject.com), creating the platform for transformative change through innovations in health care financing. Dr. Moore maintains a private solo practice in family medicine in Rochester, New York, and is a clinical assistant professor with the University of Rochester Departments of Family Medicine and Community and Preventive Medicine.

Debra L. Ness, M.S., is president of the National Partnership for Women & Families. Drawing on an extensive background in health and public policy, she possesses a unique understanding of the issues that face women and families at home, in the workplace, and in the health care arena. Before assuming her current role, she served as the National Partnership's Executive Vice President for 13 years. She graduated summa cum laude from Drew University with a bachelor's degree in psychology and sociology and has a Masters of Science degree from the Columbia University School of Social Work. She is a member of the Board of Directors and chairs the Consumer Advisory Council of the NCQA, the nation's leader in accrediting and developing quality measures for managed care organizations. She is on the Board and is Vice Chair of the Consumer Council of the NQF, established by the President's Advisory Commission on Consumer Protection and Quality in the Health Care Industry to implement a national strategy on quality protections. She sits on the Board of the Leapfrog Group, which identifies problems and proposes solutions to improve hospital systems. She serves on the Public Advisory Group on Health Care Quality of JCAHO. She is on the Steering Committee of the Ambulatory care Quality Alliance (AQA) and was recently appointed to the HQA/AQA Quality Alliance Steering Committee formed in August 2006 by HHS Secretary Leavitt, and she serves as the co-chair of the Cost/Price Transparency Working Group. Additionally, she serves on the Executive Committee of the Leadership Conference on Civil Rights (LCCR) and co-chairs the LCCR's Health Care Task Force.

W. Allen Schaffer, M.D., F.A.C.P., was former chief clinical officer for CIGNA and senior vice president of clinical strategy and health policy. He led a team that helped develop CIGNA's clinical public policy and was responsible for articulating the company's initiatives to improve health outcomes, ensure patient safety, and provide integrated patient-centered health benefits. He also served as privacy officer for CIGNA HealthCare and was responsible for advocacy outreach and external clinical relationships. Dr. Schaffer received his medical degree in 1975 from the University of Washington in Seattle, where he was granted early admission and received both medical thesis honors and the Robert H. Williams Medical Research Award.

He served his residency training at the Tulane Service of Charity Hospital in New Orleans and at Baptist Memorial Hospital in Memphis. He has held clinical faculty appointments in the Departments of Medicine at the University of Connecticut School of Medicine and at the University of Louisville School of Medicine. A fellow of the American College of Physicians, Dr. Schaffer has been published in a number of medical and professional journals, including the *New England Journal of Medicine* and the *Annals of Internal Medicine*. He currently serves on the board of the Jacobs Institute of Women's Health and the Bazelon Center for Mental Health Law. He has previously served on the boards of NCQA, the American Association of Health Plans, and the National Advisory Board for the Agency for Heathcare Research and Quality (AHRQ).

John Toussaint, M.D., is the CEO of ThedaCare Inc. ThedaCare is comprised of 4 hospitals and 21 clinics as well as other components of care including home care, hospice, seniors, and behavioral health. ThedaCare partners with local employers to decrease their targeted healthcare spend, bringing on-site innovative solutions to directly manage their costs. ThedaCare serves a seven-county region. Dr. Toussaint is an internist who has served multiple roles at ThedaCare including chief of the medicine department to chief medical officer. He has been president and CEO of ThedaCare, since March of 2000. He has been responsible for introducing the ThedaCare Improvement System which is derived from the Toyota Production system. This model of continuous improvement is transforming ThedaCare to the same level of quality performance only achieved by manufacturing companies. He is past chairman of the Wisconsin Collaborative for Healthcare Quality, which has been responsible for publicly reporting and improving performance in healthcare organizations in Wisconsin since 2003. Presently, he is the chairman of the Wisconsin Health Information Organization, a public private partnership centered on reporting provider efficiency using a centralized claims database derived from the major payers in the state. He has recently been appointed to Governor Doyle's e-Health and Patient Safety Board. ThedaCare's work has been featured in many publications some of which include *The Wall Street Journal*, *Modern Healthcare*, and *Health Management Technology*. He received his B.S. in chemistry from Cornell College in 1978, M.D. from the University of Iowa in 1982, and Internal Medicine residency from the University of Iowa, Iowa Methodist program in 1985. He has served as a adjunct professor at UW Medical School and resides in Appleton, Wisconsin.

INSTITUTE OF MEDICINE STAFF

Rosemary A. Chalk[†] is director of the Board on Children, Youth and Families (BCYF) and also serves as director of the Committee on Redesigning Health Insurance Performance Measures, Payment, and Performance Improvement (PPPI) Programs at the IOM. She has been a senior staff member of the IOM and the Division on Behavioral and Social Sciences and Education of the National Academies for almost 19 years, directing studies on vaccines and immunization finance, educational finance, family violence, child abuse and neglect, and research ethics. She took on the role of BCYF director in September 2003 and began directing the PPPI project in April 2005. For 3 years (2000 to 2003), Ms. Chalk was a half-time study director at the IOM and also directed the child abuse/family violence research area at Child Trends, a nonprofit research center in Washington, D.C., where she conducted studies on the development of child well-being indicators for the child welfare system. Over the past decade, Ms. Chalk has directed a range of projects sponsored by the William T. Grant Foundation, the Doris Duke Charitable Foundation, the Carnegie Corporation of New York, The David and Lucile Packard Foundation, and various agencies within the U.S. Department of Health and Human Services. Earlier in her career, Ms. Chalk was a consultant and writer for a broad array of science and society research projects. She has authored publications on issues related to child and family policy, science and social responsibility, research ethics, and child abuse and neglect. She was the first program head of the Committee on Scientific Freedom and Responsibility of the American Association for the Advancement of Science from 1976 to 1986 and is a former section officer for that organization. She served as a science policy analyst for the Congressional Research Service at the Library of Congress from 1972 to 1975. She holds a bachelor's degree in foreign affairs from the University of Cincinnati.

Karen Adams, Ph.D., M.T. (A.S.C.P.),[‡] was a senior program officer at the IOM. She was lead staff member on the Performance Measurement and Pay for Performance Subcommittees of the IOM's congressionally mandated study Redesigning Health Insurance Performance Measures, Payment, and Performance Improvement Programs. Her prior work at the IOM includes serving as study director of the Committee on Priority Areas for National Action: Transforming Health Care Quality and co–study director of the 1st Annual Crossing the Quality Chasm Summit: A Focus on Communities. Before joining the IOM, she held the rank of assistant professor in the De-

---

[†]Served through July 2006.
[‡]Served through February 2006.

partment of Medical and Research Technology, University of Maryland School of Medicine, and was also academic coordinator of the undergraduate medical technology program. She received an undergraduate degree in medical technology from Loyola College, a master's degree in management from the College of Notre Dame, and a doctorate in health policy from the University of Maryland. During her doctoral studies she was awarded an internship at AHRQ, during which she researched more than 30 years of innovations in medical informatics. She is also certified as a medical technologist by the American Society of Clinical Pathologists.

Samantha M. Chao, M.P.H., is senior health policy associate for the IOM's Board on Health Care Services. She completed a master's degree in health policy with a concentration in management at the University of Michigan School of Public Health. As part of her studies, she interned with the American Heart Association, where she helped develop the association's position on pay for performance. She also worked with the Michigan Department of Community Health to promote the study of chronic disease and disease prevention. Ms. Chao is currently developing a Forum on the Science of Health Care Quality Improvement and Implementation at the IOM to better understand and enhance recognition of the need for such research.

Tracy A. Harris, D.P.M., M.P.H., joined the IOM's Board on Health Care Services in 2004 as a program officer. Her work background includes clinical experience and health policy work. Previously, she was trained in podiatric medicine and surgery and spent several years in private practice. In 1999, Dr. Harris was awarded a Congressional Fellowship with the American Association for the Advancement of Science. She spent 1 year working in the U.S. Senate on many issues, including elder fraud, telemedicine, a national practitioners data bank, health professional shortage areas, stem cell research, and malpractice caps. While earning a master's degree, she worked on various projects, including Medicaid disease management and the uninsured. She has a doctor of podiatric medicine degree from the Temple University School of Podiatric Medicine and a master of public health degree with a concentration in health policy from The George Washington University.

Dianne Miller Wolman, M.G.A., most recently codirected a 3-year study on the consequences of uninsurance, which produced a series of six reports: *Insuring Health*. Before that she directed the study that resulted in the IOM report *Medicare Laboratory Payment Policy: Now and in the Future*, released in 2000. She joined the IOM's Health Care Services Division in 1999 as a senior program officer. Her previous work experience in the health field was varied, focusing on finance and payment in insurance programs.

She previously worked for the General Accounting Office, where she was a senior evaluator on studies of HCFA and its management capacity. Previously, she was a policy specialist at a national association representing nonprofit providers of long-term care services. Prior to that she held positions in policy analysis and management with the office of the secretary, U.S. Department of Health and Human Services; with a peer review organization; with a governor's task force on access to health care; and with a third-party administrator for very large health plans. In addition, she was policy director for a state Medicaid rate-setting commission. She holds a master's degree in government administration from the Wharton Graduate School, University of Pennsylvania.

Index